Human Abdominal Hydatidosis

Ajaz Ahmad Malik · Shams ul Bari

Human Abdominal Hydatidosis

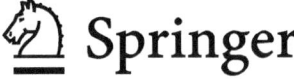 Springer

Ajaz Ahmad Malik
Department of Surgery
Sheri-Kashmir Institute of Medical Sciences
(SKIMS)
Srinagar
Jammu and Kashmir
India

Shams ul Bari
Department of Surgery
Skims/Skims Medical College
Srinagar
Jammu and Kashmir
India

ISBN 978-981-13-2151-1   ISBN 978-981-13-2152-8   (eBook)
https://doi.org/10.1007/978-981-13-2152-8

Library of Congress Control Number: 2018964082

This Springer imprint is published by the registered company Springer Nature Singapore Pte Ltd.
The registered company address is: 152 Beach Road, #21-01/04 Gateway East, Singapore 189721,
Singapore

Dedicated to our
Parents and our
Families

Preface

Although hydatid disease has got a global distribution, yet it is endemic in several parts of the world which include Mediterranean countries, North Africa, Middle-East, Indian sub-continent, Northern China, Philippines. However due to increased travel, physicians and surgeons may encounter this disease sporadically. The clinical features of liver hydatid depend on the size, number, vitality and stage of development of cyst. The diagnosis of liver hydatid cyst is established by Para-clinical investigations, especially imaging techniques such as ultrasonography, conventional radiology, and computed tomography as well as by immunological studies. Although treatment options of hydatid disease of liver have increased over the last two decades, including medical treatment, percutaneous drainage or combination of two modalities, surgery remains mainstay of the therapy. Many surgeons have tried laparoscopic intervention for hydatid cyst of liver and have had results comparable to open surgery, with added benefits of minimally invasive surgery.

The book presents an up to date review of the medical and surgical management of human abdominal hydatidosis. The publication comprises of various topics discussing the background, parasitology, epidemiology, etiology, pathogenesis, presentation, latest management and treatment of hydatid disease of liver, spleen and kidney in human beings. The book also comprises a chapters on primary peritoneal hydatidosis and minimal access management of abdominal hydatid disease.

The book will be of academic interest to all the students of medicine both undergraduates and post graduates and a reference book for teachers, academicians and researchers. The main benefit of reading this book is that since this disease entity is common in this part of world, all the relevant and latest information regarding this disease has been published in a comprehensive form which will be helpful to the researchers and students.

Jammu and Kashmir, India

Ajaz Ahmad Malik
Shams ul Bari

Contents

About the Authors

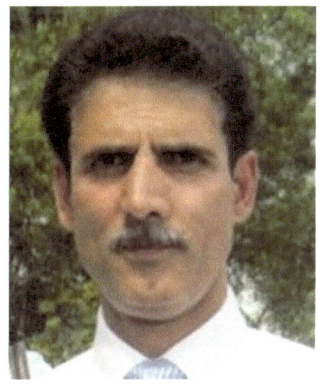

Ajaz Ahmad Malik completed his postgraduation training in the specialty of general surgery from SKIMS Srinagar, in which he subsequently joined as a faculty member in 1998. He is presently working as Professor and Division Head in the Department of General and Minimal Invasive Surgery SKIMS, Srinagar, India. He has more than 100 publications in various national and international journals to his credit and has delivered numerous lectures in various national conferences. He has contributed chapters in several books of national and international repute. He is a Fellow of International College of Surgeons (FICS), Fellow of Indian Association of Gastrointestinal Endoscopic Surgeons (FIAGES), Fellow of Minimal Access Surgery, Ganga Ram Hospital, New Delhi, India (FMAS), and Fellow of American College of Surgeons(FACS). He is a coinvestigator of an ICMR-sponsored project on Hydatid Disease in Kashmir. He is an executive editor of JMS journal and is also on editorial and reviewer board of several reputed journals.

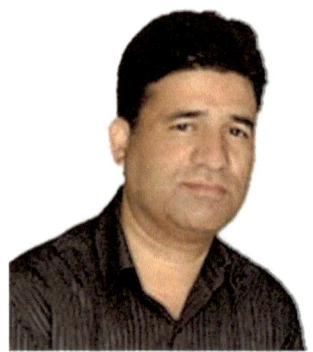

Shams ul Bari completed his postgraduation training in the speciality of general surgery from SKIMS Srinagar. He is presently working as an Associate Professor in the Department of Surgery, Skims Medical College, Srinagar, India. Earlier he worked as a consultant at Government Gousia Hospital, Srinagar. He has more than 60 publications in various national and international journals to his credit and has delivered numerous lectures in various national conferences. He has contributed chapters in several books of national and international repute. He is a Fellow of International College of Surgeons (FICS) and Fellow of Indian Association of Gastrointestinal Endoscopic Surgeons (FIAGES). He is a member of the editorial board of World Journal of Gastroenterology, World Journal of Gastrointestinal Surgery, member of the International Editorial Board IBIMA Publishing, USA, and many other journals. He is also on the reviewer board of several international journals.

Biology of the Echinococcus

Hydatid disease, also known as echinococcosis, is a parasitic infestation that has a worldwide distribution. The term "hydatid" is from the Greek word meaning a drop of water or "watery vesicle". The word "echinococcus" means "hedgehog berry". Hydatid disease was alluded to by Hippocrates around 400 BC. Its parasitic nature was hypothesized by Pallas in 1766. The history of hydatid disease and human infections with other helminths was reviewed in the 1990s and the basic life cycle of the hydatid parasite (colloquially known as a tapeworm) was finally elucidated by Groove (1990). Human cystic echinococcosis is caused by the larval stage of *Echinococcus granulosus* or *E. multilocularis*. Humans are only the accidental intermediate hosts in the life cycle of the Echinococcus. The infection is acquired by humans and other intermediate hosts after the ingestion of vegetables, fruits, and drinking water contaminated by eggs excreted by infected carnivores along with the feces, or by the handling of infected pet dogs (Milicevic 2005).

Parasitology

Echinococcosis (hydatid cyst disease) is a zoonotic parasitic infection caused by the larval stage (metacestode) of *Taenia echinococcus* belonging to the genus Echinococcus, family Taeniidae, family order cyclophyllidea, and class cestode. In the genus Echinococcus (family Taeniidae) 16 species and 13 subspecies were originally described; however, molecular studies have led to the recognition of only four clinically important species—*E. granulosus*, *E. multilocularis*, *E. oligarthus*, and *E. vogeli*. The disease in humans is called hydatidosis and the organism mostly responsible for the disease in humans is *E. granulosus*. *E. granulosus* causes unilocular or cystic hydatidosis in humans, while *E. multilocularis* is responsible for alveolar hydatid disease, also known as alveolar echinococcosis. *E. vogeli* causes a less common polycystic form of hydatid disease (D'Alessandro et al. 1979), while there is no confirmed involvement of *E. oligarthus* in human

© Springer Nature Singapore Pte Ltd. 2019
A. A. Malik, S. Bari, *Human Abdominal Hydatidosis*,
https://doi.org/10.1007/978-981-13-2152-8_1

beings. *E. felidis* and *E. shiquicus* have recently been identified as two new species, but not much is known about their pathogenicity in humans.

Echinococcus granulosus and Its Life Cycle (Fig. 1)

The life cycle of Echinococcus typically involves two hosts. The definitive host of *E. granulosus* is the domestic dog and some other related carnivores such as wild dogs, wolves, and foxes. The adult worm lives in the small intestine of these definitive hosts. It remains attached to the villi of the ileal mucosa of the definitive host for about 1 year. The adult tapeworm is 3–6 mm in length. It has a head (scolex), neck, and three to five segments. The transverse diameter of the head is 0.3–0.5 mm and it has a retractile rostellum at the end. On the head there are as many as 50 hooklets, in two circular rows, and fourqq suckers. These hooklets help in attaching the adult tapeworm to the ileal mucosa. The body is segmented into reproductive units called proglottids (Fig. 2). The adult worm is a hermaphrodite with reproductive ducts opening at a lateral genital pore. The genital pore is a common opening, but its position may vary with respect to species and strain. The first one or two segments are immature, but the last segment is disproportionally large in size and acts like a uterus; it dilates after fertilization when the eggs are fully developed; this terminal segment is gravid and contains male and female gonads and as many as

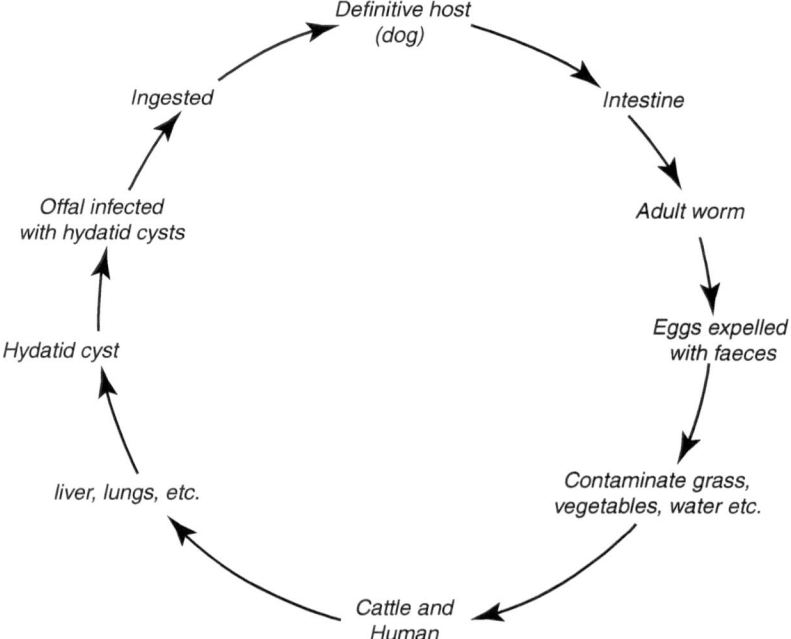

Fig. 1 Diagrammatic representation of life cycle of *E. granulosus*

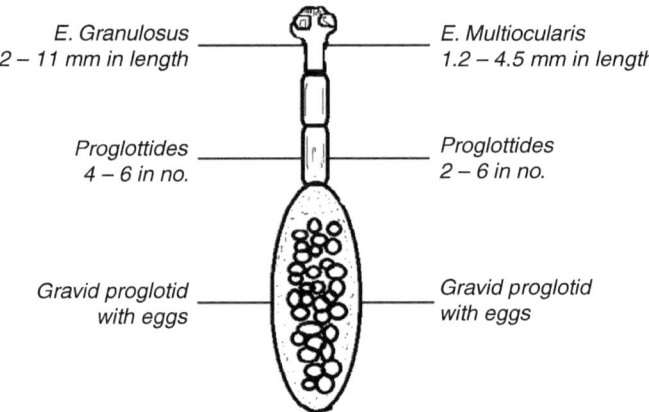

E. Granulosus
2 – 11 mm in length

E. Multiocularis
1.2 – 4.5 mm in length

Proglottides
4 – 6 in no.

Proglottides
2 – 6 in no.

Gravid proglotid
with eggs

Gravid proglotid
with eggs

Fig. 2 Adult worm of Echinococcus

5000 eggs. The eggs are ovoid in shape with an embryo inside, known as a hexa-canth, which is surrounded by several envelopes. The eggs are morphologically indistinguishable from those of other tapeworms of the genus Taenia. The metaces-tode is the second larval stage and consists of a bladder with an outer acellular lami-nated layer and an inner nucleated germinal membrane (Milicevic 2005).

During the life time of the adult tapeworm, the gravid segments detach every 7–14 days and disintegrate in the alimentary tract of the definitive host, releasing thou-sands of eggs. In the definitive host the eggs are passed into the exterior along with the feces, where they contaminate grass and vegetables grown at ground level. A dog may pass several thousand eggs daily and as many as 120 million eggs every week. These eggs are very resistant to environmental changes and can withstand extreme changes in temperature. The eggs survive and are infective for several weeks at lower temperature ranges (4–15 °C), but are very sensitive to desiccation and high tempera-tures (60–80 °C). Segmentation starts while the ovum is still in the terminal segment of the adult worm, and finally an embryo with six hooks develops within the egg. This is known as the oncosphere or hexacanth embryo (Lewall 1988).

These eggs containing embryos are ingested by grass-grazing animals such as sheep, goats, cows, buffaloes, horses, and other cattle, which then act as intermedi-ate hosts. Humans are only an accidental intermediate host. Humans usually become infected by the ingestion of contaminated vegetables and water or by direct contact with infected dogs, which usually occurs during childhood and is probably the most important route. The gravid segments of *E. granulosus* are usually found in the feces of dogs. These gravid segments can accumulate in the perineal region of dogs and disintegrate there only to release eggs. These eggs are carried by the dog's tongue to different parts of its body. Any person handling or playing with infected dogs can contaminate his or her hands and thereby become infected.

After the egg is ingested by a suitable intermediate host, the egg shell dissolves and the oncosphere is released from its surrounding envelopes. In the human duodenum the bile salts activate the hexacanth. The oncosphere attaches to and penetrates the mucosa of the intestinal wall with the help of its hooklets and reaches the lamina propria within 30–120 min after hatching. The oncospheres enter the portal circulation and are carried to the liver. The most common habitat is the liver, followed by the lungs, where the parasite develops into a larval stage—the hydatid cyst, which is the clinical presentation of *E. granulosus* infection (Milicevic 2005). Some of these cysts escape the hepatic filter and pass through the heart to the lungs and reside there only, whereas other cysts may enter the systemic circulation and reach other organs. Within the hydatid cyst large numbers of viable protoscoleces develop. From these protoscoleces, adult worms develop in the intestines within 5–7 weeks and the cycle is repeated. The life span of the adult is not known, although some have reported a life span of 2 years. This type of cycle, which includes a definitive and an intermediate host, is the sexual cycle and the resulting disease is known as primary echinococcosis. Sometimes new hydatid cysts may develop, from any of the elements of the larval stage of the parasite, in the same intermediate host, as is seen after the rupture of a hydatid cyst into the peritoneal cavity. This rupture of the main cyst into the peritoneal cavity, followed by the growth of multiple hydatid cysts in the peritoneal cavity, is known as secondary echinococcosis (Milicevic 2005).

E. multilocularis and Its Life Cycle

E. multilocularis is a small cestode, 1.2–4.5 mm in size (Fig. 2). The life cycle is the same as that of *E. granulosus*, except that the adult worm lives in the jejunum of the definitive host. Definitive hosts include domestic dogs and cats, wild rodents, and wild carnivores such as the red fox. The adult worm is characterized by fine proglottids, which reside in the jejunum of the definitive host, where gravid proglottids release eggs that are passed in the feces. Humans and intermediate hosts become infected by the ingestion of embryonated eggs. Humans can become infected either via direct contact with definitive hosts, or indirectly through food or water contaminated with eggs, or while skinning foxes (Morris and Richards 1992). The major risk of infection in humans occurs when a hunter-prey relationship is established between domestic dogs or cats and wild rodents. The domestic dogs and cats become infected by eating the rodents. In such a case, eggs in the feces of dogs and cats are the major source of infection for humans. In humans the metacestode, a larval stage of the parasite, develops in the liver and is characterized by an alveolar structure made up of several vesicles that range from <1 mm up to 15–20 cm in size. Each vesicle has a structure similar to that of an *E. granulosus* cyst (Stathatos et al. 1986). Sometimes the metacestode can grow rapidly and can cause a serious fatal disease—alveolar echinococcosis. There are no protoscoleces inside the germinative layer in alveolar echinococcosis. However, when these sterile layers are injected into a live rodent, protoscoleces are produced.

    The distribution of *E. multilocularis* is restricted to Eastern Europe, Russia, Greece, Iran, India, and some Japanese islands.

E. oligarthus and Its Life Cycle

The adult tapeworm of *E. oligarthus* is smaller in size than that of *E. granulosus*. But it has a bigger head, more hooklets, and fewer testes in the gravid segments. Geoffroy's cat, jaguars, and pumas act as definitive hosts, with rodents serving as intermediate hosts. Humans are infected only occasionally by handling wild cats; the mode of entry is via the digestive tract. The larval stage in the human liver has a multilocular character.

The species is restricted to Central and South America.

E. vogeli and Its Life Cycle

E. vogeli has a very restricted range of hosts, with bush dogs and domestic dogs acting as definitive hosts and rodents acting as intermediate hosts.

E. vogeli is also restricted to Central and South America.

Pathology of Hydatid Cyst

Cyst Stage As already discussed in the previous section, the most common habitat of *E. granulosus* is the liver, followed by the lungs, where the parasite develops into a larval stage—the hydatid cyst (Milicevic 2005). During the first 2 weeks after hatching, cellular proliferation and differentiation occurs, resulting in the formation of a vesiculated cyst, which finally develops into a metacestode. At the same time a host reaction occurs and a fibrous adventitia is formed around the cyst. However, this adventitial layer is either absent or very minimal around the cysts of *E. multilocularis*.

Development of Hydatid Cyst

Within 12 h of infestation, a small hydatid follicle may be identified in the infected organ. A well demarcated cyst is developed by the end of 1 week. At this stage local hemorrhagic extravasation and phagocytosis may occur (Lewall 1988). If the parasite survives, the number of nuclei increases, so that by the end of 2 weeks, microscopic hydatids containing fluid are formed. A hydatid cyst is visible to the naked eye by the end of 21 days. Although the growth of the cyst is even, some distortion may be seen at the sites of large ducts and blood vessels, as they act as points of resistance. The follicle attains a size of 40–50 mm at 3 months. The adventitial layer, which is the host response to the parasite, is formed by about 5 months after infestation.

Cyst Structure

Hydatid liver cysts expand slowly and asymptomatically, at the rate of about 1 mm per month or 1 cm per year, and are quite large in size at presentation. In sheep, the growth rate may be 1–5 cm per year. liver cysts located in the centre of liver are surrounded by high pressure liver parenchyma and have slow growth. Similarly, cysts located in the peritoneal cavity also show rapid growth. In *E. multilocularis*, growth is rapid, and as the peripheral growth of the cyst continues, degeneration, necrosis, and infection of the central areas of the liver can occur. In 75% of cases, a single cyst is seen, with the right and left hepatic lobes affected in 80% and 20% of cases, respectively. Although a typical hydatid cyst is unilocular, more than half are multilocular in nature.

The fully developed cyst is composed of three layers surrounding a fluid cavity (Fig. 3). The outer layer is the pericyst, also known as the adventitia or pseudocyst, the middle layer is the ectocyst or the laminated membrane, and the innermost layer is the endocyst or the germinal layer.

1. Pericyst: This layer is also known as pseudocyst or adventitia. It is an outer-most fibrous tissue layer formed by the reaction of the liver tissue to the para-site. It is present in hydatid cysts of the liver and spleen but is absent in cysts of the lung or brain. It has formed by about 5 months after infestation. This pericyst is an avascular layer and its outer layer is formed by the atrophic cells of the liver. The pericyst is an integral part of the liver and cannot be separated from the liver. There is a small capillary space between the pericyst and ecto-cyst, as a result of which the two entities can be separated from each other very easily.
2. Ectocyst (laminated membrane): this is a whitish, elastic, slimy and gelatinous layer formed by the parasite itself. It is usually 1–2 mm in thickness, but may be up to 0.5 cm thick. The laminated membrane is a mucopolysaccharide-protein-lipid complex (Richards 1984) and has a cuticular chitinous structure without nuclei. It gives some degree of rigidity to the cyst wall and is considered to be a very efficient barrier for bacteria and an ultra-filter for protein molecules.
3. Endocyst (germinal layer): this is the innermost layer, of microscopic dimensions, and is very tenuously attached to the laminated membrane. It is the only living

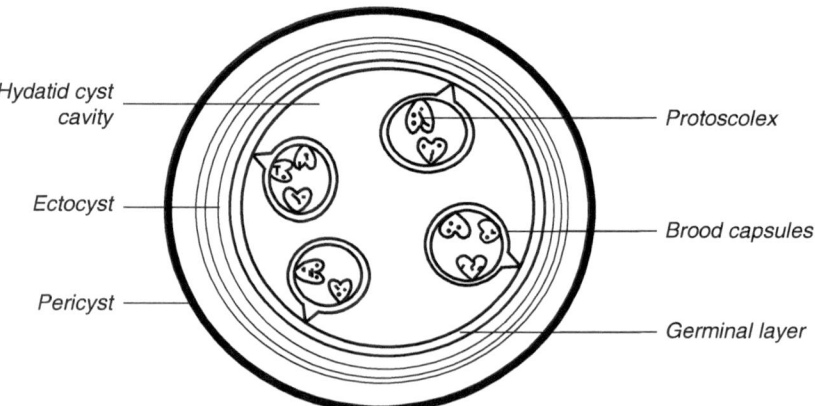

Fig. 3 Hydatid cyst of *Echinococcus granulosus*

layer of the cyst and has both secretory and absorptive functions. It is responsible for the production of the ectocyst, from outside, and crystal clear hydatid fluid, brood capsules, and scoleces and daughter cysts from inside. It has a similar structure in primary cysts, secondary cysts, and daughter cysts. The endocyst is divided into three layers. The tegument is the outermost layer and produces a laminated membrane. The middle layer is the tegumental cell region and controls the transport mechanism through the germinal membrane. The innermost layer of germinal layer known as germinal membrane has an absorptive and proliferative function and is important for the nutrition of cyst; it produces scoleces and hydatid fluid from inside. The germinal layer contains undifferentiated cells that produce invaginations toward the cyst cavity, forming brood capsules.

Hydatid Cyst Fluid Hydatid cyst fluid is actively secreted by the infecting parasite, and the progressive accumulation of hydatid fluid is a biological response to the increasing number of scoleces in the hydatid cyst. A flaccid cyst indicates a dead or degenerating cyst and a stiff cyst indicates a living cyst. The pressure in the living cyst can be as high as 100 cm of water. Due to this high intracystic pressure, explosive rupture of the cyst can occur if it is subjected to trauma or if too much manipulation is done during surgery. The hydatid fluid, which is sterile in uncomplicated cysts, is a crystal clear fluid with a specific gravity of 1.005–1.009, while the fluid is turbid in degenerated cysts. The fluid contains free scoleces; brood capsules; loose hooklets; and various salts, such as sodium chloride, sodium phosphate, sodium sulfate, and the sodium and calcium salts of succinic acid. The fluid has a pH of 6.7. Its composition is comparable to that of interstitial (extracellular) fluid. The levels of sodium, chloride, and bicarbonate are similar to those of plasma, while the potassium and calcium levels are lower than those of plasma (Vidor et al. 1986). The fluid is highly toxic and antigenic and can cause anaphylaxis. The brood capsules, free scoleces, and various salts settle at the bottom of the cyst, forming hydatid sand. One ml of hydatid fluid may contain about 400,000 scoleces. The spillage of hydatid material as a result of traumatic or iatrogenic rupture results in the implantation of protoscoleces and secondary cyst formation on the viscera. This disease in humans and animals is known as secondary hydatidosis.

Cyst Fertility

A cyst is said to be mature (fertile) when it produces the presumptive adult stage with hooks and suckers, known as the protoscolex. The protoscolex, which has four suckers and a double row of hooks, develops within the brood capsules, which are initially attached to the germinal layer by a thin stalk. As many as ten protoscoleces may develop within each brood capsule on the further proliferation of undifferentiated cells. Due to this proliferation as many as a million protoscoleces may develop within a single mature cyst of *E. granulosus*. The development of brood capsules from the germinal layer is a sign of the complete biologic development of the cyst. Old brood capsules become detached from the germinal layer and degenerate to release protoscoleces within the hydatid cavity, forming hydatid sand. In *E. multilocularis*, the brood capsules are smaller in size than those of *E. granulosus* and they generally contain only one to three protoscoleces. However, the mature stage of protoscoleces production in *E. multilocularis* rarely occurs in human beings. In *E. granulosus*, the time required to achieve maturity depends on the intermediate host. It may be up to 1 year in pigs and 1–2 years in sheep. On the other hand, in *E. multilocularis*, maturity is achieved in 2–4 months; this may reflect the short lifespan of the rodent intermediate host. On ingestion by the definitive host, protoscoleces develop into the adult stage, and thus the life cycle is completed. In the intermediate host, including human beings, each of the released protoscoleces can differentiate into a new hydatid cyst.

Daughter Cyst Formation

The development of daughter cysts is an asexual reproductive method seen in *E. granulosus*. Structurally, daughter cysts are identical to the primary cyst. Each daughter cyst has a well-developed laminated membrane and has the capacity to become fertile and produce protoscoleces within its own brood capsules developed from its germinal membrane (Richards and Morris 1990). There is a controversy regarding the exact origin of daughter cysts. It was believed that they may develop directly from the germinal layer; however, this is now considered unlikely. In vitro studies have shown that it was possible to produce cysts from ruptured brood capsules (Rogan and Richards 1986). It is now accepted that protoscoleces released from old ruptured brood capsules develop into daughter cysts (Richards and Morris 1990). However, not all the protoscoleces and brood capsules released into the hydatid cavity develop into daughter cysts—the reason being that the intact and viable germinal layer has an inhibitory effect and does not allow the development of daughter cysts. Once the cyst becomes old, the degenerated germinal membrane, with reduced power to produce capsules, loses this inhibitory property and thereby allows second-generation asexual reproduction. Any type of injury may induce daughter cyst formation, but the most common noxious agent in humans is infection and this daughter cyst formation is considered a defense reaction. The formation of daughter cysts is known as a process of endogenic vesiculation. In certain strains of the parasite and in some hosts, such as horses, the germinal membrane may be non-fertile and may not produce any brood capsules or protoscoleces. Such cysts are known as parasitologically sterile hydatid cysts, but are rarely seen in human beings. Such cysts may die and the germinal membrane degenerates. The hydatid fluid is resorbed and finally the cyst wall becomes calcified.

In *E. multilocularis*, on the other hand, the laminated membrane is thin and the pericyst is absent; this allows extensive endogenous and exogenous proliferation of the germinal layer, giving rise to a network of cellular protrusions that infiltrate the surrounding tissues. The ectogenic vesiculation becomes fulminant in the liver parenchyma and gives rise to multiple vesicles in all directions. The infected parenchyma has a multilocular appearance. Over a period of time, necrosis starts in the center of the cyst and the cyst takes the form of a spongy mass, comprising irregular cavities filled with gelatinous fluid. The process resembles a slowly growing mucoid liver carcinoma. In the majority of patients liver insufficiency occurs and the disease can prove fatal (Milicevic 2005). Furthermore, cells from the germinal layer of these protrusions can detach and be distributed via lymph or blood and can give rise to distant foci. These are known as "satellite hydatid cysts" and are characteristic of *E. multilocularis* infections (Eckert et al. 1983).

Immunobiology

Recent advances in the characterization of parasite antigens have made possible the immunodiagnosis of hydatid disease in both humans and domestic animals. The antibody response to infection has formed the basis of several immunological tests. The sources of hydatid antigens are the cyst fluid, germinal membrane, protoscoleces, and the walls of the brood capsules. Higher concentrations of antigens have been seen in the cysts in humans and in sheep as compared with antigen concentrations in the cysts in cattle and pigs. Higher antigen concentrations are found in hepatic cysts and lower concentrations are seen in pulmonary cysts (Musiani et al. 1978). Studies have revealed that the cysts of *E. multilocularis* are a poor source of antigens as compared with the cysts of *E. granulosus*. Several antigens specific to the parasite have been found in hydatid fluid.

The immunobiology of both the adult worm and the cyst stage has been extensively studied (Heath 1986). Two important immunoreactive antigens have been studied extensively. Both are lipoproteins with a small carbohydrate moiety; they have been named antigen A (also known as antigen 4) and antigen B (also known as antigen 5). The exact locations of these antigens have been studied by indirect immunofluorescence and by electron microscopy (Davies et al. 1978). In addition to hydatid fluid, these antigens have been found in other structural components of hydatid cysts. Antigen A has been identified in the inner portion of the germinal layer, the walls of brood capsules, and in the sub-tegumentary cells of protoscoleces, while antigen B has been identified in the tegumentary cells of the anterior part of the protoscoleces, in the germinal layer, and in the laminated membrane.

Both antigen A and antigen B leak from the hydatid cysts and elicit the production of IgG and IgE antibodies in the host. It has been found that these antibodies have no effect on the growth and development of cysts. Once there is infestation with Echinococcus, there is depletion of complement, particularly during the rapid growth of *E. multilocularis* (Ciobanca and Junie 2011; Lewall and McCorkell 1986). Several studies have revealed that the laminated membrane plays an important role in immunoprotection and the host IgG readily binds to the laminated membrane, thereby forming a barrier to the host immune cells (Heath and Lawrence 1976).

The cyst fluid of *E. granulosus* contains a heat-stable low-molecular-weight cytotoxic agent that is able to cross the cyst wall and interfere with the immunocompetent cells of the host (Morris and Richards 1992), thereby resulting in immunosuppression. The host lymphoid cells, which are in close contact with the laminated membrane, are often necrotic. This can cause depletion of T cells and can increase the metastatic proliferation of *E. multilocularis* (Baron and Tanner 1976).

The Human Body's Immune Response to Echinococcosis

Echinococccus granulosus

The immune response to *E. granulosus* involves both cellular and humoral immunity. In the early stage, a cell-mediated response involving macrophages, neutrophils, and eosinophils is established. Both Th1 and Th2 responses develop. Elevated levels of Th1 cytokines, especially interferon-G (IFN-G), have been seen, as well as elevated levels of Th2 cytokines, such as interleukin (IL)-4, IL-5, and IL-6 (Stathatos et al. 1986). The reason for both the Th1 and Th2 responses is not yet known. It is presumed that the complex antigenic organization of Echinococcus may stimulate both T-cell subsets. Th1 and Th2 responses usually down-regulate each other with a cross-inhibitory mechanism (Morris and Richards 1992). After treatment (chemotherapy/surgery), the Th2 response quickly drops and the Th1 response becomes predominant (Davies et al. 1978). The metacestode has a complex protective response to the host immune response. It minimizes the host reaction by exposing several immunomodulatory molecules to its host, interfering with the complement system, altering leukocyte function, or using molecular mimicry (Davies et al. 1978)

Echinococcus multilocularis

The *E. multilocularis* parasite induces a strong cellular immune response. Cellular immunity viaTh1 cytokines plays a crucial role in defense against the parasite. IL-12 seems to be a key factor in the induction of the Th1 profile. In the liver, lesions appear to be surrounded by large granulomas consisting of macrophages, T-lymphocytes, and myofibroblasts. The Th2 response has been associated with disease exacerbation, and IL-4/5 has been detected in patients with progressive disease. Several mechanisms have been proposed to explain the *E. granulosus* avoidance of the host immune response, including molecular mimicry, immunomodulation, and antigen and DNA polymorphism (Musiani et al. 1978).

Epidemiology and Incidence

Although hydatid disease has a worldwide distribution, it is relatively common in sheep-rearing areas of the world. The disease is endemic in Australasia, South America, the Middle East, the Far East, and South Africa (Eckert et al. 1983). The disease is rare in Western Europe and the United States. Both sexes and all age groups are affected with equal frequency. The disease is more prevalent in rural areas with poor sanitation facilities and poor living conditions, where human beings, dogs, and cattle exist in close proximity. The distribution of the disease is influenced by the presence of dogs, mostly if they are allowed to remain loose and have access to uncooked viscera. Data from rural areas where Echinococcus is endemic also shows variation in the number of dogs infected. In the Niger Delta, 85% of dogs are infected; in Morocco, 58.5%; in the central region of Wales, 25%; and in western isles (island on the west coast of Scotland) 10% of dogs are infected. Differences have also been found between rural, urban, and semiurban dog populations where dogs are fed raw offal either deliberately or inadvertently, and the offal may be infected. In very remote areas dogs may feed on the dead bodies of intermediate hosts, including human beings, thereby resulting in transmission of the parasite. Eggs shed from infected hosts are exposed to a large number of extrinsic factors that have an effect on egg survival; humidity is the most important factor. Although the eggs can remain viable for up to 12 months, their infectivity declines with age. It has been found that the egg life span is inversely proportional to temperature. Dispersion of the eggs is achieved by the movement of the proglottids after they are shed and also by animals, birds, and insects. Infection of the intermediate host depends on the availability, density, and infectivity of the eggs and on the feeding patterns of the host. However, the final number of cysts that become established is determined by the natural and acquired resistance of the host to infection.

At present no global data on the actual incidence of human hydatidosis is available; the incidence is established with respect to surgically treated patients or chemotherapy data obtained from hospital records. In endemic areas the incidence depends on the level of health care and veterinary control. Annual incidence rates vary widely. In eastern Australia the incidence is 0.57 per 100,000 population per year; in Greece there are 13 cases per 100,000 persons (Morris and Richards 1992); in Cyprus 9.3 per 100,000 persons (Polydorou 1980); and in Yugoslavia 3.8 per 100,000 persons (Morris and Richards 1992). In Iran 0.5% of all hospital admissions are for hydatid disease (Amir-Jehad et al. 1975). The incidence is also increasing in non-endemic areas because of the upsurge of emigration and trade. Occupation and culture have a marked influence on the incidence of hydatid disease. The higher incidence of hydatid disease in rural areas as compared with urban areas is a result of farming activities, particularly in sheep-rearing areas. In northern America, hydatid disease is limited to hunters and fur trappers, particularly those dealing with fox fur. In Lebanon, it used to be the case that shoemakers showed a higher incidence of hydatid disease compared with other occupations, as they used to prepare leather using dog feces mixed with water (Schwabe and Abou-Daoud 1961). Also, the incidence in Lebanon is higher in the Christian than in the Muslim community, as the Christian community tends to have a closer association with dogs. In New Zealand the prevalence is higher in Maoris than in the European population because of their closer association with dogs.

Organs Involved

The larval form of Echinococcus can invade any organ system and the distribution of the infection is limited by the blood flow. Hydatid cysts can occur in the liver, lungs, spleen, brain, muscle, bone, spinal cord, heart, orbit, and peripheral arterial system. The liver is the most common site for hydatid cysts and is involved in 75% of cases. Milicevic (2005) followed by the lungs in 15%, kidneys in 5%, muscles in 5%, bones in 3%, spleen in 2–3%, orbit in 1–2%, and brain in 0.2–2.4%. The heart accounts for 1–1.5% of cases and 60% of these are found in the left ventricular myocardium. The central nervous system, particularly the brain, accounts for 0.2 to 2–4% of cases and 60% of these are found in children aged less than 15 years Zinner et al. (1997).

References

Amir-Jehad AK, Faria R, Furzad A. Clinical echinococcosis. Ann Surg. 1975;182:541–6.
Baron RW, Tanner CE. The effect of immunosuppression on secondary *Echinococcus multilocularis* infection in mice. Int J Parasitol. 1976;6:37–42.
Ciobanca PT, Junie ML. Serological diagnosis and its applicability to the prophylaxis and therapy of hydatid cyst in human patients. Sci Parasitol. 2011;12(1):39–46.
D'Alessandro A, Rausch RL, Cuello C, Aristizabel N. *Echinococcus vogeli* in man, with a review of polycystic hydatid disease in Colombia and neighbouring countries. Am J Trop Med Hyg. 1979;28:303–17.
Davies C, Rickard MD, Bout DT, Smyth JD. Ultra structural immunocytochemical localization of two hydatid fluid antigens (antigen 5 and antigen B) in the brood capsules of ovine and equine *Echinococcus granularis* and *Echinococcus multilocularis*. Parasitology. 1978;77:143–52.
Eckert J, Thompson RCA, Mehlhorn H. In: Thompson RCA, editor. Proliferation and metastases formation of larval Echinococcus and hydatid disease. London: Allen and Unwin; 1983. p. 250–84.
Groove DI. A history of human helminthology. Oxford: C.A.B. International; 1990.
Heath DD. Immunobiology of echinococcus infections. In: Thompson RCA, editor. The biology of echinococcus and hydatid disease. London: Allen and Unwin; 1986. p. 165–88.
Heath DD, Lawrence SB. *Echinococcus granulosus*: development in vitro from oncosphere to immature hydatid cyst. Parasitology. 1976;73:417–23.
Lewall DB. Hydatid disease: biology, imaging and classification. Clin Radiol. 1988;53:863–74.
Lewall DB, McCorkell SJ. Rupture of echinococcal cysts: diagnosis classification and clinical implications. Am J Roentgenol. 1986;146:319–94.
Milicevic MN. Hydatid disease. In: Blumgart LH, Fong Y, editors. Surgery of the liver and biliary tract, vol. 2. China: WB Saunders; 2005. p. 1167–97.
Morris DL, Richards KS. Hydatid disease; current medical and surgical management. Oxford: Butterworth-Heinemann; 1992.
Musiani P, Piantelli M, Lauriola L, Arru E. *Echinococcus granulosus*: specific quantification of the two most immunoreactive antigens in hydatid fluids. J Clin Pathol. 1978;31:475–8.
Polydorou K. The control of echinococcus in Cyprus. FAO World Ann Rev. 1980;(33):19–25.
Richards KS. *Echinococcus granulosus* equinus: the histiochemistry of the laminated layer of the hydatid cyst, vol. 22; 1984. p. 21–32.
Richards KS, Morris DL. Effect of albendazole on human hydatid cysts: an ultra-structural study. Hepatobiliary Surg. 1990;2:105–13.

Rogan MT, Richards KS. In vitro development of hydatid cysts from posterior bladders and rup-
   tured brood capsules of equine *Echinococcus granulosus*. Parasitology. 1986;92:379–90.
Schwabe CW, Abou-Daoud K. Epidemiology of echinococcosis in the Middle East. Am J Trop
   Med Hyg. 1961;10:374–81.
Stathatos C, Kontaxis A, Zaphiracopoulos P. Hydatid cyst of the liver. Sixth Panhellenic Congress
   of Surgery VI. 1986. p. 365.
Vidor E, Piens MA, Abbas M, Petavy AF. Biochemie du liquid hydatique. Ann Parasitol Hum
   Comp. 1986;61:333–40.
Zinner MJ, Schuxirtz SI, Ellis H. Liver abscess and hydatid disease, Maingot's abdominal opera-
   tions, vol. II. 10th ed. Stamford, CT: Appleton and Lange; 1997. p. 1513–44.

Hydatid Disease of the Liver: Clinical Presentation and Complications

Clinical Features

The clinical presentation of hydatid disease of the liver depends on several factors which include location and the size of cyst, the stage of development and whether the cyst is alive or dead. The majority of patients with hydatid liver disease have indolent presentation in an otherwise healthy individual. Almost 75% of patients are asymptomatic, and hydatid cyst is detected as an accidental finding during a routine examination (Barnes and Lillemoe 1997). The cyst is usually more than 5 cm, when symptoms do occur. In symptomatic patients, the most common complaint is the dull aching pain in the right upper quadrant (80%) followed by dyspepsia and vomiting in 50% of patients. Diaphragmatic pain can be seen in cysts protruding from the superior surface of the liver.

Some patients may present only once there is some complication. Acute abdominal pain with fever is seen in patients with hydatid rupture, biliary complications and secondary bacterial infection. Patients with biliary rupture may develop cholangitis with subsequent fever, rigours and jaundice. The most common physical finding is the right upper quadrant mass or hepatomegaly as seen in 70% of patients followed by right upper quadrant tenderness in 20% of patients. Rarely, patients with hydatid liver cysts develop polyarthritis secondary to increased levels of IgE. Sometimes an infected child harbouring a large cyst becomes cachectic, "hydatid cachexia" (MiLicevic 2000; Dawson et al. 1988).

Jaundice is an important clinical feature of patients with hydatid disease. There are five likely reasons for jaundice in patients with hydatid liver disease (Morris and Richards 1992).

(a) *Intraductal debris*: In patients where there is a cysto-biliary communication, daughter cysts and hydatid membranes will migrate into the biliary tract. This can result into obstruction of the duct followed by jaundice, cholangitis and even the liver abscess. If the patient has cholangitis, intravenous antibiotics and intravenous fluids should be started immediately. This should be followed by

© Springer Nature Singapore Pte Ltd. 2019
A. A. Malik, S. Bari, *Human Abdominal Hydatidosis*,
https://doi.org/10.1007/978-981-13-2152-8_2

ERCP with papillotomy to remove the cysts and membranes from the ducts. If nonoperative method fails, patient will need a common bile duct exploration to clear the CBD at the time cystectomy.

(b) *Compression by cyst*: A large hydatid cyst placed centrally may also cause jaundice by extrinsic compression of bile ducts. In majority of the cases, jaundice is relieved once the cyst is removed. In some cases it may persist due to fibrosis. Some patients may need a biliary stent, while others may need a biliary enteric bypass.

(c) *Sclerosing cholangitis*: This is an extremely serious and well-established late complication seen in those patients who have underwent hydatid cyst surgery, and surgeons have used any of the available scolicidal agents. The cysto-biliary communication may be seen in as many as 5–30% cases, and improper use of such toxic agents may result into caustic damage of the biliary tree, leading to sclerosing cholangitis. It is because of this that most of the authors do not recommend injection of scolicidal agent into the unopened cyst. The cavity should be opened and contents removed, cavity cleaned meticulously and searched for any biliary communication before using any of the available scolicidal agents. The role of systemic steroids in managing this situation is being studied. Balloon dilatation with stent placement and biliary enteric bypass are the various methods attempted to manage this problem.

(d) *Drug induced*: Patients put on albendazole therapy can develop hepatocellular dysfunction with the subsequent jaundice (Morris and Smith et al. 1987). If therapy is not stopped immediately, severe hepatocellular necrosis can occur. In view of this fact, all patients put on albendazole therapy should undergo liver function tests every 2 weeks. The rising level of enzymes is an indication of liver toxicity.

(e) *Alveolar echinococcus infection* caused by *Echinococcus multilocularis* is another reason for jaundice as it causes a lethal disease with destruction of the liver.

Complications

More than 30% of patients harbouring hydatid disease of the liver present with complications (Barnes and Lillemoe 1997). Infection or suppuration of the cyst and rupture of the hydatid cyst into the biliary tree are the most common complications seen in clinical practice. In addition to these, the other complications may also be seen, which include rupture into the peritoneal cavity, rupture into the pleural cavity, internal rupture, rupture into hallow viscera and rupture into vascular system. Rarely external compression may be seen leading to portal hypertension. We have come across complications in as many as 26% patients. Out of these, infection was seen in 14.49% of patients, rupture into the biliary tract in 8.69% of patients and intraperitoneal rupture in 2.89% of patients (Barnes and Lillemoe 1997).

Suppuration of the Hydatid Cyst Liver

The hydatid cyst which has been asymptomatic for years may present with a secondary bacterial infection with resultant pus formation. *Escherichia coli* is the most frequently isolated microbe from the pus of these infected hydatid cysts. Once there is pus formation, the parasite dies. The incidence of infected liver hydatid is variable ranging from 11 to 27% (Akinoglu et al. 1985). The patient may present with features of pyogenic liver abscess such as fever, pain in the right hypochondrium, anorexia, tachycardia and other systemic features. Since the laminated membrane has got antibacterial property, infection occurs only when the integrity of laminated membrane is lost. Contents of infected hydatid cyst are usually bile stained as the suppuration of the cysts is almost always associated with the rupture into the biliary tree (Lewall 1988). Certain structural changes are seen in the infected hydatid cyst. A thick pyogenic membrane develops on the inner surface of the adventitial layer of the hydatid cyst. As a result of this, the cyst wall becomes rigid, and the intracystic pressure increases. The infective process may also spread into the surrounding areas such as the diaphragm and viscera resulting into formation of adhesions.

Pressure Effects and Rupture of the Hydatid Cyst

Patients can present with various symptoms either due to direct pressure or distortion or rupture into the neighbouring structures including viscera and large vessels (Fig. 1). The cyst has always the tendency to grow in the direction of least resistance. In those areas where there is less space available, the growing cyst can cause serious symptoms as in the brain, while in other areas such as the liver, it can grow enormously, before it becomes symptomatic. In the liver, as the cyst enlarges, the adjacent liver tissue gets atrophied along with a corresponding hypertrophy of the remaining liver tissue (Fig. 2). In other cases enlargement of cyst can result into

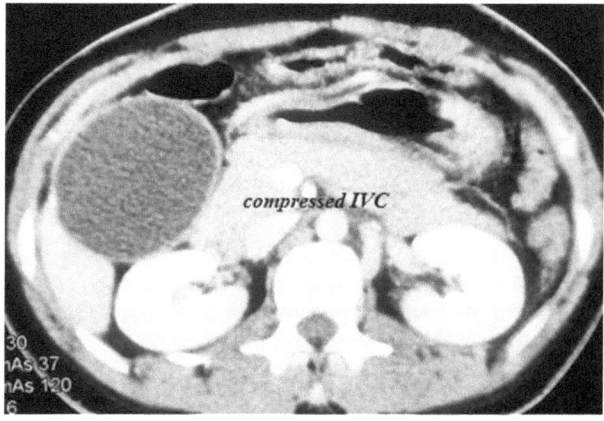

Fig. 1 Hydatid cyst in the right lobe of the liver causing compression on IVC

compressed IVC

Fig. 2 Huge hydatid cyst in the right lobe of the liver with compensatory hypertrophy of the left lobe

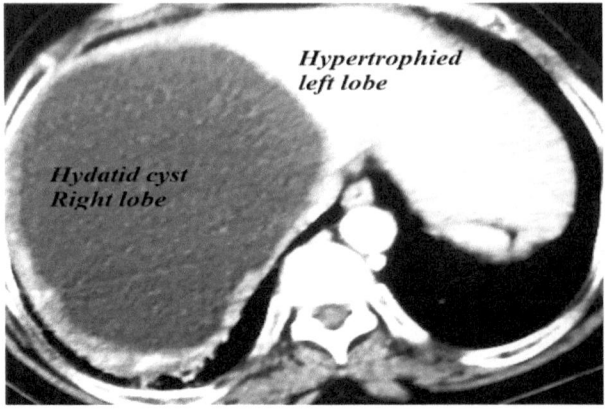

rupture of the endocyst, which is known as obscure rupture. In concomitant rupture, the contents enter bronchial or a biliary tree, while in free rupture, the hydatid contents disseminate freely into the peritoneal cavity, pleural cavity or pericardial cavity (Barnes and Lillemoe 1997).

Intrabiliary Rupture

The incidence of biliary rupture is quite variable. Erguney et al. reported low incidence of 5–10%, while Barrada et al. have reported incidence up to 25% (Zargar et al. 1992). Intrabiliary rupture could be an internal rupture or external rupture. In order to understand internal rupture, it is essential to know what is a univesicular cyst and what is a multivesicular cyst. A univesicular cyst is a single cyst with an intact laminated membrane. On the other hand, in a multivesicular cyst, there is no laminated membrane, and a large number of daughter cysts are floating in a pool of turbid yellowish fluid along with a gelatin-like amorphous material. It is not possible to differentiate a univesicular cyst from multivesicular cyst on the surface of the liver. At some stage in the past, the laminated membrane of the univesicular cyst ruptures within its own pericystic cavity, and scoleces are released, which grow over a period of time into daughter cyst. Such cysts are known as multivesicular cysts (Milicevic 2000).

As the cyst enlarges, it comes in close contact with small bile ducts. As the enlargement continues, it compresses the bile ducts causing bile stasis and increase in intraductal pressures. This increase in intraductal pressures causes fissures in the wall of ducts. Bile escapes through the breach in the wall of the duct and accumulates in the potential space between the pericyst and laminated membrane, thereby separating the two and eventually causing the rupture of the laminated membrane. The laminated membrane degenerates forming the debris. This is known as an internal rupture (Saidi et al. 1997). This type of rupture of the laminated membrane can be caused by trauma to the liver or relentless expansion of the cyst. Once there is rupture of the laminated membrane, the spilled hydatid fluid is absorbed into the circulation, thereby inducing sensitivity to the hydatid antigen. The fluid content of the cyst with ruptured laminated membrane grossly looks like a thin pus, and a secondary infection may be suspected. However, it is as sterile as a fluid in a univesicular cyst with an intact laminated membrane unless there are white cells in the fluid or bacteria are seen in gram staining.

Further increase in intracystic pressure causes pressure necrosis of the wall of the nearby major bile duct. The pressure necrosis of the wall of the bile duct creates an opening large enough to allow the escape of smaller daughter cysts and fragments of laminated membrane into the biliary tract, resulting into a cysto-biliary fistula frequently. The cyst can rupture into small-calibre ducts or large-sized ducts depending on the site of the cyst. Although in some cases rupture into the large bile duct may allow full evacuation of the cyst contents and thereby leads to a spontaneous cure, however, in majority of cases, evacuation is incomplete, and this can result into secondary infections or cholestatic jaundice with recurrent cholangitis (Al-Hashmi 1971). In endemic areas, 3–10% of cases of obstructive jaundice are due to intrabiliary rupture of hydatid cysts (El Mufti 1989). The patients with intrabiliary rupture present with a triad of symptoms which is important to understand in order to reach a diagnosis. These include biliary colic, cholangitis and jaundice due to partial intermittent or complete ductal obstruction. In addition to it, many patients will give history of passage of germinative membranes in the faeces (Hydatid enteria). In almost 90% of patients, the rupture is silent or occult. In these patients, the bile probably seeps into the cyst from eroded ducts through the disintegrating laminated membranes. Since the bile is a noxious agent, the cyst dies and may even get partly calcified, and the contents will be bile stained. No visible biliary communication is seen in such patients. Cysts located close to porta hepatis can cause obstruction by compression on CBD or CHD. In those patients who are already sensitized and there is a rapid discharge of contents into the bile ducts or into any of the body cavities, anaphylaxis can occur, while in others, pruritus, urticarial rash or asthma can occur.

Intraperitoneal Rupture of Hydatid Cyst Liver

As the liver cyst grows, it follows the line of the least resistance and hence grows centrifugally towards the outer surface of the liver. The most superficial surface of the liver thins out and ultimately tears. Intraperitoneal rupture of the hepatic hydatid cyst (Fig. 3) is one of the less common complications, and its incidence varies from 1 to 4% as reported in literature (Al-Hashmi 1971). Several forms of intraperitoneal rupture have been reported in literature (El Mufti 1989).

1. Diffuse peritonitis: In acute cases of rupture, with the release of contents of the cyst into the peritoneal cavity, patients will develop features of diffuse peritonitis due to irritation of the peritoneum. Patients will have severe abdominal pain, fever, tachycardia, tenderness of the whole abdomen and even shock. Such patients need urgent resuscitation followed by immediate laparotomy. Thorough

Fig. 3 CT image showing ruptured hydatid cyst in the left lobe of the liver

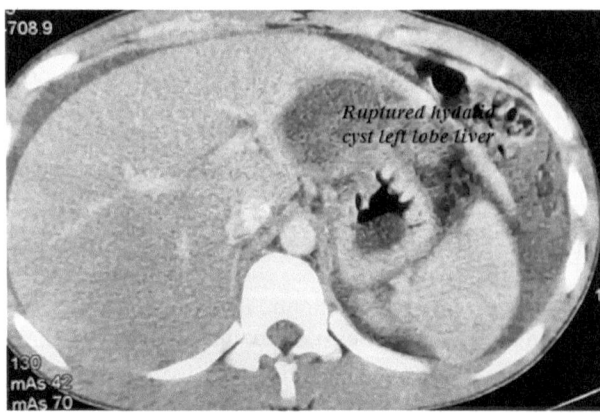

lavage of the peritoneal cavity is needed using any of the available scolicidal agents such as hypertonic saline. All the quadrants of the peritoneal cavity need a meticulous cleansing to remove debris and daughter cyst escaped into the peritoneal cavity. The cyst in the liver is managed in usual manner. Despite meticulous cleaning, the disease tends to become disseminated within the peritoneum.

2. Anaphylactic shock: Some patients with rupture of hepatic hydatid cyst may present with an anaphylactic shock. There will be generalized urticaria with a circulatory collapse, which can even prove fatal if not treated immediately.

3. Disseminated abdominal hydatidosis: In some patients following an intraperitoneal rupture, patient may present with silent abdominal distension only. In these patients usually there is slow leakage of cyst contents, both fluid and daughter cyst, into the peritoneal cavity which initially goes unnoticed. Over a variable period of time, as the leakage continues and daughter cyst increases in size and number, the abdomen starts distending, and patients feel abdominal discomfort. In some cases, distension is so much that patients can have respiratory embarrassment (Bari and Malik 2006). Once the laparotomy is done in such patients, we may find thousands of cysts spread throughout the peritoneal cavity (Fig. 4).

4. Dumb-bell hepato-peritoneal cyst formation: It is a very rare type of intraperitoneal rupture of hepatic hydatid cyst. As the cyst enlarges in size, the pericyst thins out, and a small tear develops in it, through which a laminated membrane herniates. The laminated membrane remains intact, but it grows outside the liver as a pouch. Thus there will be two cysts, one is inside the liver and other is outside the liver. Both the cysts remain intact giving the appearance of a dumb-bell. The cyst which is inside the liver remains small, while the cyst outside the liver attains a large size. This can mimic ascites, and if aspiration is attempted, it can lead to anaphylaxis.

The intraperitoneal rupture although less common is a life-threatening complication of hydatid cyst of the liver (Sherlock 1981; Wani et al. 2005; Wani et al. 2011). The protoscoleces, brood capsules and daughter cyst released into the peritoneal cavity have the potential of growing into a mature hydatid cyst. As already

Fig. 4 Silent and massive abdominal distension due to disseminated abdominal hydatidosis following trauma

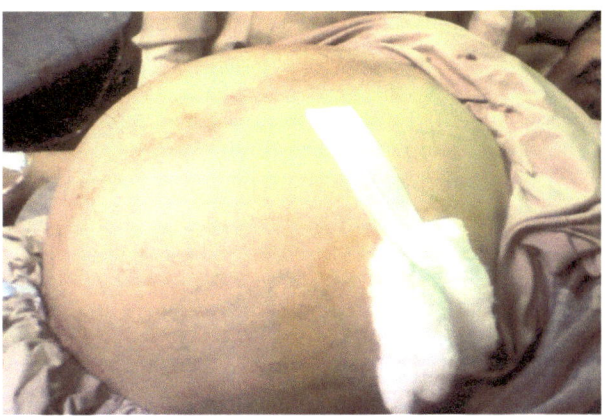

mentioned, patient can present with ascites, intestinal obstruction and massive abdominal distension. The process is quite slow, and the patient can remain asymptomatic for years after the rupture of the cyst. This is the asexual life cycle of *Echinococcus* and is seen only in the intermediate host. This asexual cycle is also known as secondary echinococcosis.

Intrathoracic Rupture

The rupture of hydatid cyst of the liver into the thoracic cavity is an uncommon complication, and its incidence has been reported from 0.6 to 16% in the literature (Gomez et al. 1995; Aletras et al. 1971). The hydatid cyst located in the upper and posterior parts of the liver tends to grow in a cephalic direction. Continuous and relentless pressure on the diaphragm pushes the liver cyst into the chest cavity. Initially a sympathetic pleural effusion occurs which is sterile, and lots of adhesions develop between the liver and diaphragm. As the cyst goes on increasing in size, the muscular diaphragm is stretched and ultimately eroded by the liver cyst. This process is usually clinically silent, or the patient may have a vague chest pain or a shoulder pain, dry cough and dyspnoea. As the intracystic pressure increases, the cyst ruptures, and if adhesions have formed already, the rupture remains localized and abscess formation is there. This abscess may communicate with the liver cyst by a narrow opening. The combination of infection and pressure causes destruction of lung parenchyma with a resultant pneumonitis and lung abscess. In rare cases the cyst may have a free rupture into the pleural cavity, resulting into empyema of pleural cavity. In such cases the pleural cavity may be filled with hydatid debris and large number of daughter cyst (hydatopiothorax). The hydatid cyst may sometimes erode into a bronchiole, and in such cases, patients may have severe cough, and they can cough out hydatid membranes and daughter cysts. By the time the final rupture occurs, the diaphragm has usually become attached to both the liver and the lung. The symptoms are of a sudden tearing pain, dyspnoea and anaphylactic shock from which the patient may die. After recovery, chest radiograph shows a pleural effusion or a pyopneumothorax particularly if the rupture into the pleura occurred after rupture into the bronchus. If the contents of the cyst are bilious because of communication with a bile duct, sputum will be bile-tinged, and this a pathognomonic sign of bronchobiliary fistula (Amin et al. 2007).

Rupture of a cyst into the pleural cavity necessitates emergency thoracotomy. The objectives of the operation are to remove the parasite, drain the hepatic cavity and re-expand the lung immediately. Separate drainage of the chest is necessary. The type of operation usually performed is pleurectomy with decortication of the lung. Even in neglected cases of rupture with pyothorax and daughter cysts in the visceral or parietal pleura, same type of operation is indicated. The danger of recurrence is greater when the cyst ruptures into the bronchi, but this danger does not justify pleuropneumonectomy. In patients where a biliary complication is suspected, exploration of the common bile duct along with T-tube drainage is mandatory. Transpleural approach is preferred by many authors (Amin et al. 2007; Avlamis and Bonelos 1961), as exposure is better and the lung complications can be dealt with more amicably. In patients with abdominal complications, either the incision can be extended to the abdomen or a separate abdominal incision can be made. It is always necessary to drain the common bile duct in a ruptured cyst with biliary complications. After dissecting the bronchial fistula, the opening in the diaphragm is enlarged and the hepatic cavity cleared and drained sub-diaphragmatically. It is important to be conservative in dealing with pulmonary complications, and in the majority of patients, lung complications are reversible. The drainage of the hepatic cavity must be continued until complete closure of the cavity occurs. The diaphragm is closed in layers, and a water seal drainage catheter is left in the pleural cavity for at least 48 h. It is important to remember that if the hydatid cyst of the liver has penetrated the diaphragm to enter the chest cavity, the lungs must be first handled in an appropriate manner through thoracotomy. The cyst in the liver can be managed through incision in the diaphragm by simply enlarging the diaphragmatic hole. The pleural space should be drained in the standard manner.

The hepatic hydatid cyst can also rupture into various other adjacent organs such as the gall bladder, stomach, duodenum, small intestine and pericardium. Patients may vomit hydatid membranes and cysts (hydatidemesis). Other patients may pass hydatid membranes and cysts in the faeces (hydatidenteria). Rupture into the pericystic vessels, gall bladder, aorta, inferior vena cava and pericardium with subsequent embolism has also been reported in the literature.

References

Akinoglu A, Bilgin I, Erkocak EU. Surgical management of hydatid disease of liver. Can J Surg. 1985;28:171–4.
Aletras H, Dadoukis J, Aidonopoulos A. Bronchobiliary fistulas. Galenus. 1971;13:657–63.
Al-Hashmi HM. Intrabiliary rupture of hydatid cyst the liver. Br J Surg. 1971;58:228–32.
Amin MU, Tahir A, Akhtar MS. Transdiaphragmatic rupture of huge hepatic hydatid cyst with formation of bronchopleural fistula. J Coll Physicians Surg Pak. 2007;17(7):431–2.

Avlamis G, Bonelos K. Problems and surgical treatment of broncho-biliary fistulas due to hydatid cyst of the liver. Second Panhellenic Congress of Surgery. 1961;II:960–4.

Bari SU, Malik AA. Delayed diagnosis of traumatic rupture of hydatid cyst liver. Int J Surg. 2006; https://doi.org/10.1016/ijsu.

Barnes SA, Lillemoe KD. Liver abscess and hydatid cyst disease. In: Schwasy Z, Ellis, editors. Maingot's abdominal operations, vol. 2. 10th ed. Stamford, CT: Apleton and Lange; 1997. p. 1513–44.

Barnes SA, Lillemoe KD. Maingot's abdominal Operations. Liver abscess and hydatid cyst disease, vol. 2. 10th ed. Stamford, CT: Apleton and Lange; 1997. p. 1513–44.

Dawson JL, et al. Surgical treatment of hepatic hydatid disease. Br J Surg. 1988;75:946–50.

El Mufti M. Surgical management of hydatid disease. London: Butterworths; 1989.

Gomez R, Moreno E, Loinaz C, De la Calle A, Castellon C, Manzanera M, Herrera V, et al. Diaphragmatic or transdiaphragmatic thoracic involvement in hepatic hydatid disease: surgical trends and classification. World J Surg. 1995;19(5):714–9. https://doi.org/10.1007/BF00295911.

Lewall DB. Hydatid disease: biology, imaging and classification. Clin Radiol. 1988;53:863–74.

MiLicevic MN. Hydatid disease. In: Blumgart LH, Fong Y, editors. Surgery of liver and biliary tract. 3rd ed. London: W. B. Saunders Company; 2000.

Morris DL, Richards KS. Hydatid disease: current medical and surgical management, vol. 167. Jordon Hill, Oxford: Butterworth-Heinemann; 1992. p. 1197.

Moris DL, Smith PG. Albendazole in hydatid disease -hepatocellular toxicity. Transactions R Soc Trop Med Hyg. 1987;81(2):343–4.

Saidi F. A new approach to the surgical treatment of hydatid cyst. Ann R Coll Surg Engl. 1997;59:115–20.

Sherlock S. Hydatid disease: disease of liver and biliary system. Oxford: Blackwell Scientific; 1981. p. 247–452.

Wani RA, Malik AA, Chowdri NA, Wani KA, Naqash SH. Primary extrahepatic abdominal hydatidosis. Int J Surg. 2005;3:125–7.

Wani NA, Kosar T, Gojwari T, Robbani I, Choh NA, Shah AI, Khan AQ. Intrabiliary rupture of hepatic hydatid cyst: multidetector-row CT demonstration. Abdom Imaging. 2011;36(4): 433–7. https://doi.org/10.1007/s00261-010-9675.

Zargar SA, Khuroo MS, Khan BA, Dar MY. Intrabiliary rupture of hydatid cyst: sonographic and cholangiographic appearances. Gastrointest Radiol. 1992;17:41–5.

Diagnosis of Hydatid Disease of the Liver

The diagnosis of uncomplicated hydatid cyst or any of its complication rests on a strong clinical suspicion. History and clinical examination remain the mainstay of diagnosis of hepatic hydatid disease. The history of having resided or travelled in an endemic area is always a strong diagnostic lead. Despite the extent of lesion, the patient is generally healthy because of the absence of any systemic ill effects of echinococcal disease.

In view of very slow growth of cyst, the patients hardly give history of acute pain, rather they give a history of a vague discomfort in the right hypochondrium. Accidently an asymptomatic mass is palpated in the right hypochondrium in patients where the large cyst is located on the inferior aspect of the liver. The history of sudden urticaria along with a mild abdominal pain following a trauma or fall suggests the possibility of rupture of hydatid cyst. Rarely, patients with hydatid liver cysts develop polyarthritis secondary to increased levels of circulating IgE levels and immune complexes.

Laboratory Evaluation

Laboratory evaluation of patients with hydatid liver disease reveals non-specific data. The white blood cell count is elevated if the cyst is infected; otherwise it is usually within normal limits. Eosinophilia of more than 3%, although seen in 35–45% of patients, is non-specific in endemic areas where other parasitic infestations are seen. In patients where the cyst has ruptured into the biliary tree, there can be a transient elevation of GGT or ALP along with eosinophilia (>500/ml) and hyperamylasaemia. When the cyst ruptures, the level of eosinophilia increases markedly (Akinoglu et al. 1985; Al-Hashmi 1971).

© Springer Nature Singapore Pte Ltd. 2019
A. A. Malik, S. Bari, *Human Abdominal Hydatidosis*,
https://doi.org/10.1007/978-981-13-2152-8_3

Immunological Diagnosis of Hydatid Disease

Several immunodiagnostic tests have been used for the diagnosis of hydatid disease. These include Casoni skin test, complement fixation test (CFT), indirect haemagglutination (IHA), indirect immunofluorescence antibody test (IFAT), immunoelectrophoresis (IEP), counterimmune electrophoresis, double-diffusion test (DD), radioallergosorbent test (RAST) and latex agglutination test (LA). However, tests such as enzyme-linked immunosorbent assay (ELISA) or immunoblotting have been found to be more specific and sensitive and are now widely used (Milicevic 2000). In certain groups of human population and in young children, antibody response may be low, resulting into a false-negative test. False-positive results have also been reported, especially in patients suffering from other helminthic disease due to cross infection and in patients with tumours. Several antigens have been extracted from different sources for eliciting antibody response and for use in serological diagnosis. The most frequently used antigen has been the hydatid cyst fluid, which contains the mixture of antigens derived from the host and parasite. Two major parasite antigens have been derived from the hydatid fluid. One is antigen B (Ag B), which is a thermostable antigen (Oriol et al. 1971), and antigen 5 (Ag 5), which is a heat-unstable antigen (Pazznoli et al. 1975). Both antigen B and antigen 5 are lipoproteins and are among the most specific native antigens used for immunological diagnosis of hydatid disease. Antigen 5 occurs in the inner part of the germinal layer, brood capsules and protoscoleces, while antigen B is found in tegumental cells mainly and in laminar and germinal layers to some extent. Although antibody response involves all the immunoglobulins such as IgM, IgG, IgA and IgE, IgG is the most important and can persist for several years even after the surgical removal of hydatid cysts. Various secondary tests such as identification of IgG subclass are available for detection of antibody and for increasing the specificity. Similarly tests like immunoblotting are used to demonstrate the reactivity of serum antibodies with subunits of *E. granulosus* antigens. Since the hydatid cyst often remains localized, the absence of a positive echinococcal serology does not rule out the disease (Barmes and Lillemoe 1997).

The Casoni skin test was used in the past to evaluate patients suffering from echinococcal disease. This test consists of injecting a sterilized hydatid cyst fluid subcutaneously. The patients sensitized to echinococcal antigens will develop a wheal with multiple pseudopodia and erythema at the injection site within half an hour (early positive reaction), while in others, erythema and oedema will develop after 24 h (late positive reaction). Sensitivity of 80% and specificity of 70% have been seen with this test (Barmes and Lillemoe 1997). A major drawback of the test is that the test remains positive for several years even after the infection has been eradicated. The test may also be falsely positive in carcinomatosis, teniasis and leishmaniasis. False-positive results occur due to poor standardization of the protein antigens in the test kits. False-negative tests have been observed in infected cyst, in calcified cyst and in children as the intensity of immune reaction depends on the amount of absorption of antigen (Barmes and Lillemoe 1997). It has been found that the test may sensitize the patient to echinococcal antigens and may cause anaphylaxis in those patients who have high levels of circulating echinococcal IgE. In view of above disadvantages and availability of various other serological tests, Casoni test is no longer used for diagnosis of echinococcal disease (Matosian 1983).

Serum immunoelectrophoresis is currently the most reliable procedure and has the sensitivity of 90%. The indirect haemagglutination (IHA) has a sensitivity of 85%, while compliment fixation (CFT) has a sensitivity of 70%. Enzyme-linked immunosorbent assay (ELISA) has a sensitivity of more than 90% and has an advantage of its low cost and ability to automate the procedure (Milicevic 2000).

These serological tests have little value during follow-up of patients after surgery or who have been put on chemotherapy. Ideally the titters should fall after surgery, and rising titters should indicate recurrence. The serum immunoelectrophoresis has got high specificity and remains positive for 6–12 months after surgery, while IHA remains positive for several years after surgery. Although IHA is very sensitive, but false positive test may occur in infection with *T. solium*. The CFT has some role in monitoring of patients after treatment as it reverts to negative only 6 months after surgery or death of a parasite (Lainer et al. 1987). Another serological test known as an arc 5 double-diffusion test is a simple test based on antigen-antibody precipitation.

ELISA in combination with ultrasound abdomen is quite useful for population surveys in endemic areas. In ELISA, an anti-immunoglobulin reagent labelled with one of several enzymes is used, which produces a colour change with a substrata (Farag et al. 1975). Specific immune complexes and specific antibodies can be detected by ELISA.

Several tests have been introduced in clinical practice for rapid diagnosis of the disease. One such test is human basophil degranulation test. It has a sensitivity of almost 90% and becomes negative only 1 week after surgery. Serological tests for *Echinococcus multilocularis* are not as sensitive as for *E. granulosus*, although recently excellent results have been obtained with Western blot analysis (Milicevic 2000).

Radiology

The asymptomatic patients with hydatid disease are often diagnosed after an abnormality is detected on X-rays or scans in a patient who is being evaluated for some other reason. The plain X-ray of the abdomen is not of any help as the radiodensity of noncalcified cysts is the same as that of the rest of the liver (Pedrosa et al. 2000). Standard radiographic examination reveals calcification in the liver in about 50% of patients with a calcified or dead cyst. The calcification is curvilinear or ring like and involves pericyst. Daughter cysts may also calcify and produce several rings of calcifications. However calcification does not necessarily indicate death of parasite. In endemic areas, elevation of the right hemidiaphragm in an otherwise healthy asymptomatic patient is highly indicative of hydatid liver. Occasionally a fluid level will be seen when there is a communication of a cyst with the gastrointestinal tract (Pedrosa et al. 2000).

Ultrasonography

Ultrasonography (US) is a simple, readily available, cheap and non-invasive diagnostic technique. US detects almost 90% of hydatid liver cysts. Abdominal ultrasound is the investigation of choice as it defines the number, site, dimensions and viability of cysts. US not only detects the characteristics of cyst but also its relation to biliary tree and biliary vessels particularly the hepatic veins. Ultrasound is also useful for evaluating treatment options. It can easily differentiate cystic lesion from non-cystic lesion and univesicular and multivesicular cysts. The daughter cysts have a characteristic appearance within the main cyst cavity and look like radiating spokes of a wheel— known as **cartwheel sign** (Morris and Richard 1992; Saidi 1997). Ultrasonography is a very useful investigation in patients with suspicious rupture of hydatid cyst into the biliary tract as it can easily differentiate between gallstones and daughter cysts. However, it cannot accurately localize the position of cyst in the liver substance so as to plan the proper surgical exposure. The ultrasound can be used for screening of patients in endemic areas and among family members. It is an ideal modality used for following the natural course of hydatid cystic disease. The natural course of hydatid cyst disease can be divided into two stages, and each stage has its characteristic ultrasonography appearance. During the proliferative stage of the disease, as the cyst grows, it attains a smooth, well-defined univesicular shape. This stage is known as a simple noncomplicated cyst. As the biological development continues and involution occurs, the cyst becomes fully mature, which looks like a cellular mass and has a germinal membrane with brood capsules arising from it.

On the basis of ultrasonographic features, hydatid cyst of the liver has been grouped into five types by Hassen Gharbi (Gharbi et al. 1981), which correspond to the evolutionary stages of the hydatid cyst (Figs. 1, 2 and 3). These are:

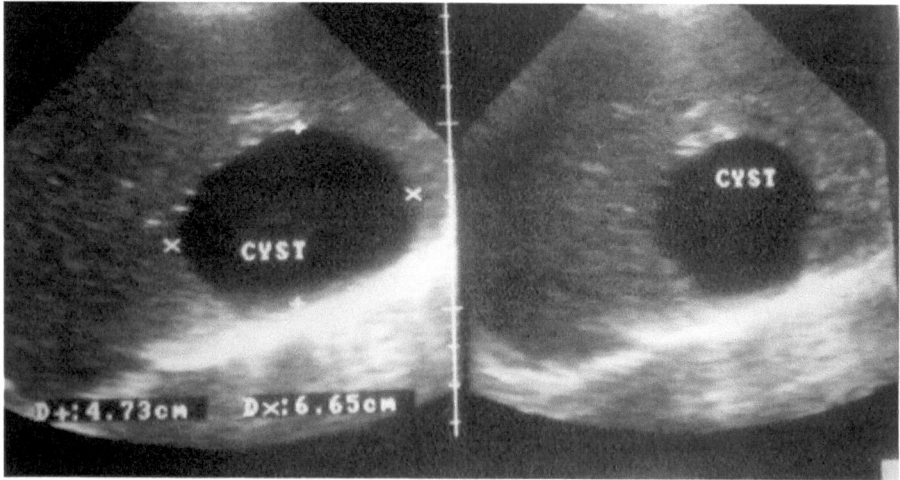

Fig. 1 USG picture showing Type 1 hydatid cyst

Fig. 2 USG image of
Type 111 hydatid cyst

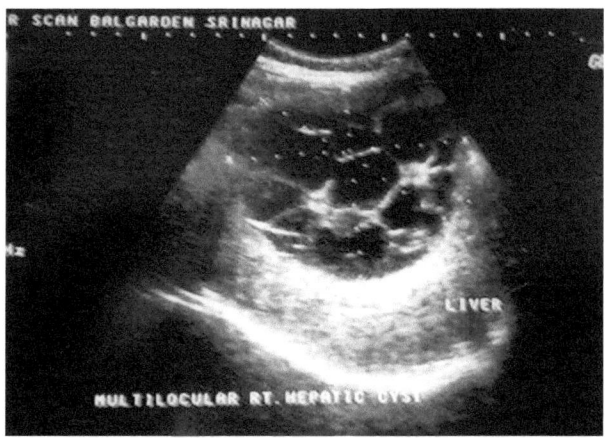

Fig. 3 USG image
showing two hydatid cyst
cavities in the right lobe of
the liver

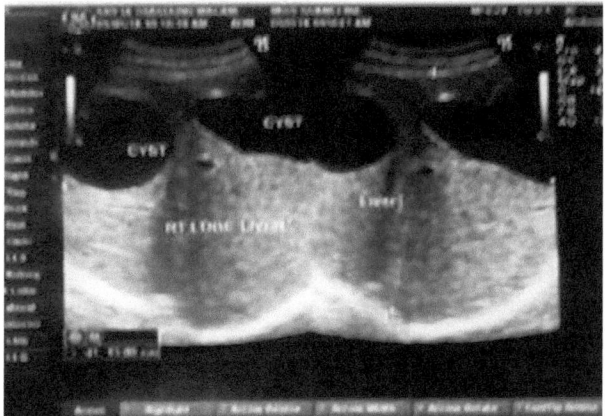

1. Type I—pure fluid collection with a thin wall
2. Type II—fluid collection with a split wall/detached membrane (water lily sign)
3. Type III—cystic lesion with multiple septa and daughter cysts (honeycomb appearance)
4. Type IV—cyst with heterogeneous appearance
5. Type V—cyst with reflecting thick walls

This ultrasonography classification has been further modified into four types (Beggs 1985), which is based on the natural course of hydatid disease.

• **Type 1**: The simple hydatid cyst; it is a young hydatid cyst and on US is a well-circumscribed cyst with a well-defined cyst wall. These cysts can have a budding signs on the germinative membrane of the endocyst or may contain a hydatid sand which is best demonstrated by changing the position of the patient. Hydatid sand is seen as a hyperechogenic foci floating freely in the cystic fluid. These two signs are important for differentiating hydatid cyst from other benign cysts.

- **Type 1A**: In this we find an undulating hyperechogenic membrane (detached germinative) which floats in the cystic fluid (water lily sign).
- **Type 11**: A characteristic rosette appearance is seen due to presence of daughter and granddaughter cysts.
- **Type 111**: The cyst is filled with an amorphous mass and has a solid and or semi-solid appearance. This can lead to a diagnostic problem and may be considered wrongly as a tumour, liver abscess or haemangioma. Presence of calcification in the wall of the cyst and hypoechogenic lacunar structures seen in the matrix helps in diagnosis.
- **Type 1V**: The cyst is completely calcified and has an egg shell appearance.

With the aim of updating old Gharbi classification, the WHO in 2001 has devised a standardized USG classification system for classifying a hepatic hydatid cyst. It is used to assess the stage of hepatic hydatid cyst on ultrasound and is useful in deciding the appropriate management for it depending on the stage of the cyst (Giorgio et al. 2009).

- **CL:** It is a unilocular anechoic cyst without any internal echoes and septations and the cyst wall not visible.
- **CE 1:** It is an anechoic cyst with fine and uniform echoes settled in it which represents hydatid sand, cyst wall visible.
- **CE2:** Cyst which is multivesicular and multiseptated with daughter cysts, giving an appearance of rosette or honeycomb. This is the active stage of the cyst.
- **CE3**: Unilocular cyst with daughter cysts and detached floating laminated membranes giving appearance of a water lily sign. This is the transitional stage of the cyst.
- **CE4:** Cysts with heterogeneous degenerative contents and no daughter cysts, giving an appearance of a ball of wool (known as ball of wool sign). It indicates degenerative nature of the cyst.
- **CE5**: Cysts characterized by a thick calcified wall; the cyst is inactive and infertile.

US can also be used as an intraoperative tool to determine the accurate site and size of the cyst and its relation to any adjacent vital structures such as vessels and ducts. Intraoperative ultrasound also helps in exact location of small non-palpable and deep-seated cysts. It also helps to look for any exogenous vesiculation and to rule out any cystobiliary communication. On USG, cystobiliary communication can be suspected if any of the following features is found such as air in the cyst, hydatid membrane or daughter cysts in the biliary tree, heterogeneous pattern of the cyst and loss of continuity of the wall of the bile duct adjacent to cyst wall.

The ultrasonography can also be used for nonoperative interventional treatment procedures and for monitoring the response in patients put on nonoperative management. Ultrasonography is also used for follow-up of patients which have been put on medical treatment. Shrinkage of cyst, membrane detachment or loss of germinal layer and cloudy appearance of intracystic fluid are signs of therapeutic effect. The USG is also used for follow-up of patients after surgery, although interpretation of residual cavities persisting after surgery is difficult (Fig. 4). Practically all residual cavities disappear by 18 months. However in children residual cavities disappear and get replaced by fibrous tissue within 6 months (Marino et al. 1995). If any cavity persists beyond 18 months, further evaluation is needed by USG monitoring and immunological tests. In all those patients whose cavities increase in size or the fluid collection increases or seropositivity is increasing, further surgical intervention may be required.

Computed Tomography

The sensitivity of computed tomography (CT) scan in detecting liver hydatid is almost 100%. CT is more sensitive than US in localizing and delineating the exact extent of the cyst (Figs. 5, 6, 7, 8, 9, 10 and 11). Daughter cysts and exogenic cysts

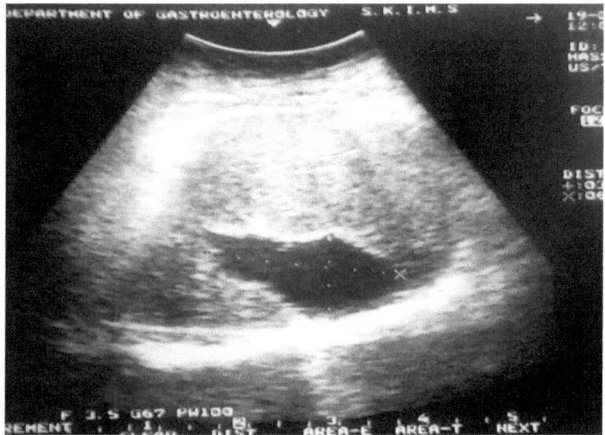

Fig. 4 USG showing residual cavity in the liver 2 months after surgery

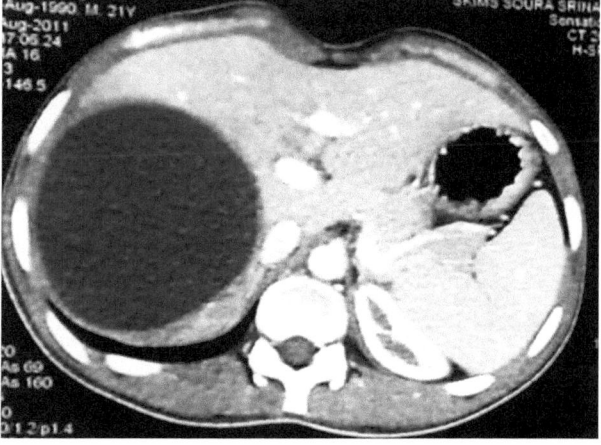

Fig. 5 CT image showing unilocular hydatid cyst of the liver

Fig. 6 CT image showing a multiloculated hydatid cyst in the liver

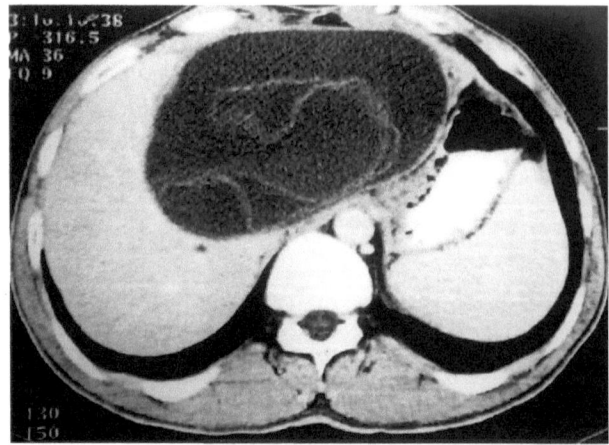

Fig. 7 CT image of hydatid cyst liver with detached membranes

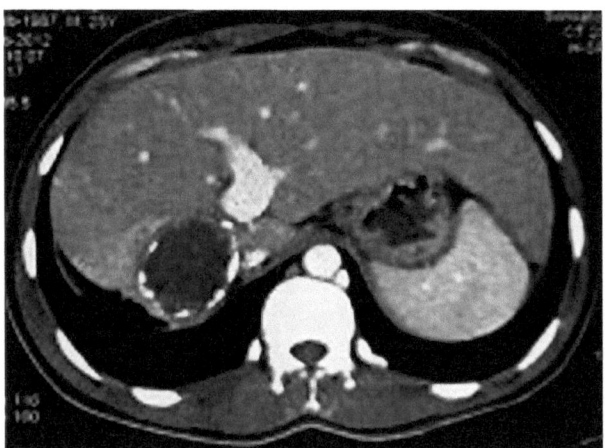

Fig. 8 CT image of hydatid cyst in both the right and left lobe

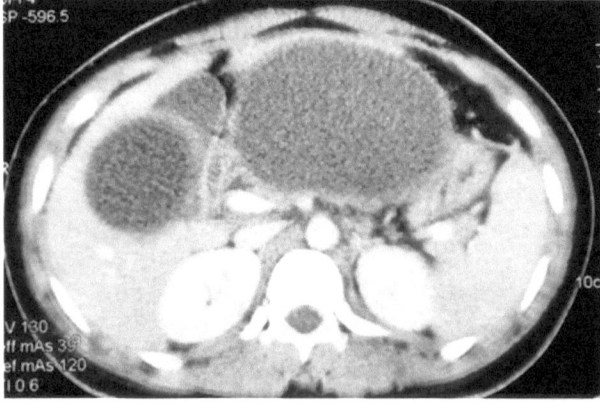

Fig. 9 Multilocular
hydatid liver with
contained rupture

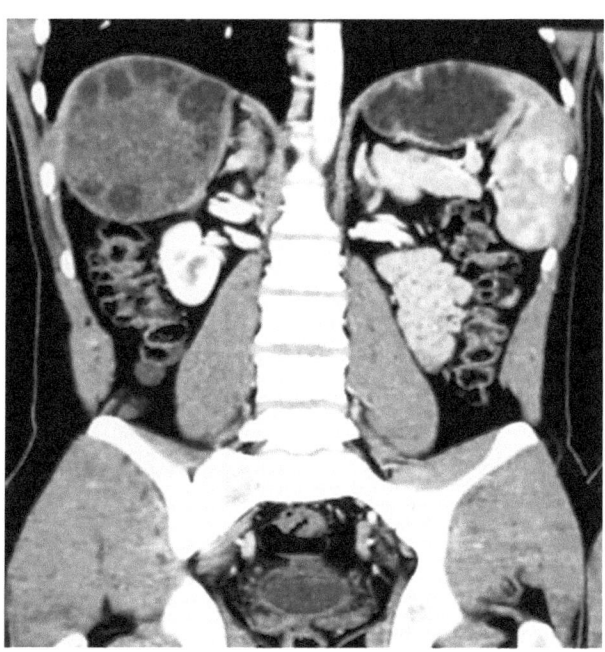

Fig. 10 Multiple
intrahepatic multilocular
hydatid cyst

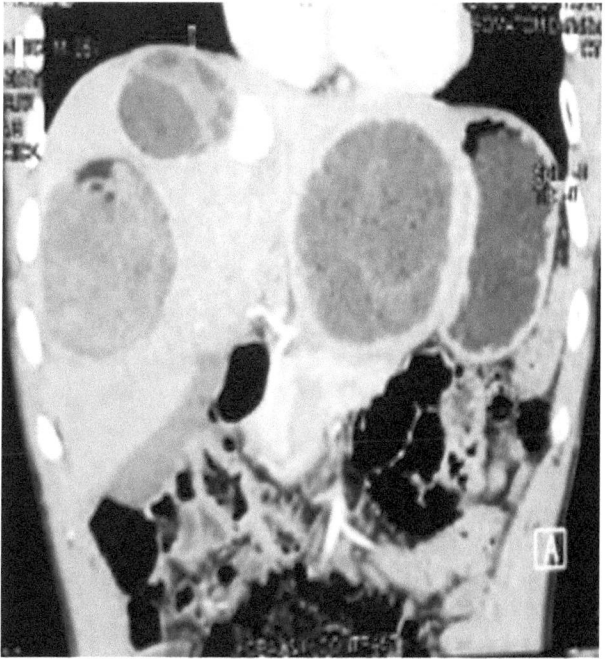

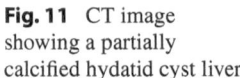
Fig. 11 CT image showing a partially calcified hydatid cyst liver

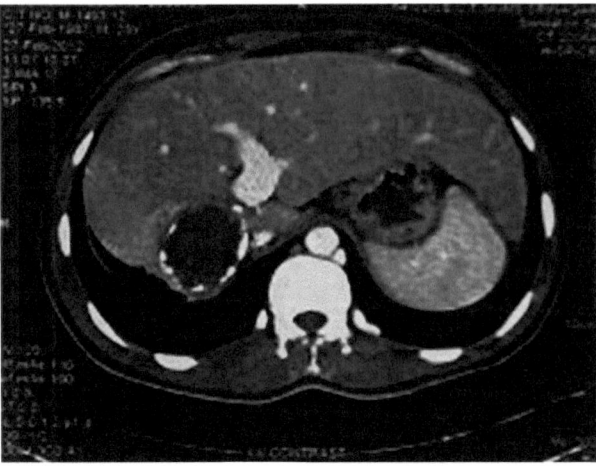

are demonstrated more accurately on CT scan. CT abdomen is considered as an essential investigation before surgery by most of the surgeons as it gives the surgeon an accurate road map regarding the location and size of cysts in the liver. CT is an investigation of choice when diagnosis is uncertain and when infection or rupture of the cyst is suspected. CT may display the same findings as are seen in ultrasonography (Pedrosa et al. 2000). A hydatid cyst on CT scan appears as a water-attenuation cyst with an attenuation value of 3–30 HU. A special value of CT scanning is the discovery of calcification of pericyst layer, which otherwise cannot be seen on USG (Fig. 11). Typically hydatid cyst is seen as a well-attenuated lesion even without calcification on CT abdomen. Detached laminated membrane from the pericyst is visualized as a linear area of increased attenuation within the cyst—**serpentine structures** (Fig. 7). The calcification of the wall of the cyst as seen in non-viable cyst is well demonstrated on computed tomography (Fig. 11) (Pedrosa et al. 2000).

On CT image, daughter cysts are seen as round structures located peripherally within the mother cyst (Fig. 6). The daughter cysts are surrounded by high-density fluid giving appearance of radiating spokes in a rosette-like pattern (Pedrosa et al. 2000). These cysts usually contain fluid with a lower attenuation than that of the fluid in the mother cyst. CT appearance of the cyst also changes in patients who are on chemotherapy, and the cyst becomes shrunken, and then density of residual cyst increases.

Magnetic Resonance Imaging (MRI)

It is a good imaging technique in patients with skeletal and vertebral disease and cardiac hydatidosis. This imaging modality is too complex and expensive for routine use. On MRI, hepatic hydatid cyst may be seen as homogeneous hypointense lesion on T1-weighted images and a homogenous hyperintense lesion on T2 images. Although non-specific, the presence of a hypointense rim at the periphery of the cyst is considered as a characteristic feature of hydatid cyst, which otherwise is not seen in nonparasitic cysts. This hypointense rim is seen in long-standing cysts and is believed to represent the outermost layer of the hydatid cyst, which is rich in collagen and is generated by the host itself. Daughter cysts on MRI are seen as cystic structures attached to the germinal layer (Pedrosa et al. 2000). These cysts are hypointense or isointense as compared to the intracystic fluid on T1-weighted images and hyper intense on T2-weighted images. Collapsed membranes of parasite are seen as twisted linear structures within the cyst at MRI. Although calcification of the wall of cyst is better demonstrated at CT, MRI is superior in depicting irregularities of the rim. Probably, this irregular rim represents the early stage of detachment of the membranes (Pedrosa et al. 2000)

Angiography

It can be used only in selected patients. It is a useful diagnostic modality but is too invasive to be used routinely. However it can be used in nonendemic areas as a supplementary diagnostic tool. The area of the cyst is seen as large area devoid of blood supply. In the late venous phase, the pericyst layer is seen as a distinctive halo around a central avascular area.

Scintigraphy

Scintigraphy is a very reliable investigation for demonstrating any space-occupying lesion in the liver which is greater than 4 cm in size. Although scintigraphy performed in anterior, posterior and lateral view is more helpful in localizing the cysts in the liver, it has not been widely accepted as a modality of investigation.

Endoscopic Retrograde Cholangiography (ERCP) and Percutaneous Transhepatic Cholangiography (PTC)

ERCP and PTC should be performed in all patients where rupture of hydatid cyst into the biliary tract is suspected, particularly in patients with obstructive jaundice. On cholangiography, the entire biliary tract can be delineated, and if the cyst has ruptured in to the biliary tree, daughter cyst and membranes can be seen in the biliary channels, thereby helping to differentiate obstructive jaundice from nonobstructive jaundice (Bekhti et al. 1977; Bari and Malik 2006; El-Mufti 1989).

ERCP is both diagnostic and therapeutic and should be done in all patients whose USG shows hydatid cyst membranes and daughter cyst in the bile ducts or in patients with jaundice (Zargar et al. 1992). ERCP with endoscopic papillotomy should be done before surgery in all those patients whose USG, CT or ERCP shows hydatid material in the common bile duct and in those with cholangitis irrespective of biliary communication (Milicevic 2000). ERCP with endoscopic papillotomy has a role in the postoperative period as well as in certain groups of patients which include patients with a high-output fistula (more than 1000 ml/24 h) and biliary fistula persisting for more than 3 weeks, in patients whose postoperative USG shows hydatid membranes or daughter cysts in the CBD and in patients with postoperative jaundice. In these patients postoperative endoscopic papillotomy can markedly reduce the postoperative morbidity and hospital stay.

References

Akinoglu A, Bilgin I, Erkocak EU. Surgical management of hydatid disease of liver. Can J Surg. 1985;28:171–4.

Al-Hashmi HM. Intrabiliary rupture of hydatid cyst the liver. Br J Surg. 1971;58:228–32.

Bari SU, Malik AA. Delayed diagnosis of traumatic rupture of hydatid cyst liver. Int J Surg. 2006; https://doi.org/10.1016/j.ijsu.2006.09.007.

Barmes SA, Lillemoe KD. Maingot's abdominal operations. Liver abscess and hydatid cyst disease, vol. 2. 10th ed. Stamford, CT: Apleton and Lange; 1997. p. 1513–44.

Beggs I. The radiology of hydatid disease. AJR Am J Roentgenol. 1985;145(3):639–48.

Bekhti A, Schaaps JP, Capron M, Dessaint JP, Santoro F. Treatment of hepatic hydatid disease with mebendazole: preliminary results in four cases. Br Med J. 1977;ii:1047–51.

El-Mufti M. Surgical management of hydatid disease. London: Butterworths; 1989.

Farag HD, Bout D, Capron A. Specific immunodiagnosis of human hydatidosis by the enzyme linked immunosorbent assay (ELISA). Biomedicine. 1975;23:276–8.

Gharbi HA, Hassine W, Brauner MW, et al. Ultrasound examination of the hydatid liver. Radiology. 1981;139(2):459–63.

Giorgio A, Di Sarno A, de Stefano G, et al. Sonography and clinical outcome of viable hydatid liver cysts treated with double percutaneous aspiration and ethanol injection as first-line therapy: efficacy and long-term follow-up. AJR Am J Roentgenol. 2009;193(3):W186–92. https://doi.org/10.2214/AJR.08.1518.

Lainer AP, Trujillo DE, Schantz PM. Comparison of serological tests from the diagnosis and follow up of alveolar hydatid disease. Am J Trop Med Hyg. 1987;37(3):609–15.

Marino JM, Bueno J, Prieto C. Hepatic hydatidosis in children. Euro J Pediatric Surg. 1995;5:274–6.

Matosian RM, Kane GJ, Chantler SM. The specific immunoglobulin in hydatid disease. Immunology. 1983;22:423.

Milicevic MN. Hydatid disease. In: Blumgart LH, Fong Y, editors. Surgery of the liver and biliary tract, vol. 2. Philadelphia, PA: WB Saunders; 2000. p. 1167–204.

Morris DL, Richards KS. Hydatid disease; current medical and surgical management, vol. 167. Oxford: Butterworth-Heinemann; 1992. p. 1197.

Oriol R, Williams JF, Perez-Essordi ML. Evaluation of purified lipoprotein antigens of Echinococcusgranulosus in the immunodiagnosis of human infection. Am J Trop Med Hyg. 1971;20:569–74.

Pazznoli R, Piantelli M, Perucci C. Isolation of the most immuno reactive antigens of Echinococcusgranulosus from sheep hydatid fluid. J Immunol. 1975;115:1459–63.

Pedrosa I, Saiz A, Arrazola J, Ferreiros J, Pedrosa CS. Hydatid disease: radiologic and pathologic features and complications. Radiographics. 2000;20(3):795–817.

Saidi F. A new approach to surgical management of hydatid disease. Am Cole Surg Engl. 1997;59:115–8.

Zargar SA, Khuroo MS, Khan BA, Dar MY, Alai MS, Koul P. Intrabiliary rupture of hepatic hydatid cyst: sonographic and cholangiographic appearances. Gastrointest Radiol. 1992;17(1):41–5. https://doi.org/10.1007/BF0188850.

Surgical Management of Hydatid Liver Disease

The mainstay of treatment of hepatic hydatid disease is surgery and is presently the only viable treatment for alveolar hydatid disease (Arif et al. 2008). Even today, controversy exists as to the extent of operation performed. Advances in management have been made with the use of newer anthelminthic and application of percutaneous aspiration in selected patients.

The goals of treatment for hepatic hydatid cyst are complete elimination of parasite, prevention of recurrence and minimizing mortality and morbidity risk. It is essential to choose the most appropriate treatment with regard to disease-specific characteristics such as number of cysts, location of the cyst, presence of cystobiliary communication, patient's condition and availability of experienced staff, experienced surgeon and an experienced interventional radiologist. Therapeutic modalities available to treat hepatic hydatid cyst include both nonoperative management and operative management.

Nonoperative Methods It includes chemotherapy and percutaneous aspiration under USG guidance.

Chemotherapy

Many drugs have been used as medical treatment in hydatid disease including antimony, arsenic, iodides and mercury. However, none of them were found to be effective. Recently the benzimidazole carbamate group of drugs has been introduced and was found effective against larval stage of both *E. granulosus* and *E. multilocularis* (Arif et al. 2008). This benzimidazole carbamate group of drugs blocks glucose uptake in the parasite and causes depletion of its glycogen stores. The drug causes death of germinal membrane cells, and the cyst loses its ability to maintain haemostasis and integrity (Heath et al. 1975).

© Springer Nature Singapore Pte Ltd. 2019
A. A. Malik, S. Bari, *Human Abdominal Hydatidosis*,
https://doi.org/10.1007/978-981-13-2152-8_4

Percutaneous Aspiration

Recently, a percutaneous drainage of hydatid cysts, popularly known as PAIR (puncture, aspiration, installation of scolicidal agent and reaspiration) technique, has been used (Khuroo et al. 2002; Arif et al. 2008). When percutaneous aspiration is combined with local and systemic administration of albendazole, cure rate is more than 60%. Percutaneous drainage is often indicated in patients with uncomplicated unilocular cysts, sick patients, patients with comorbidity and patients with multiple previous surgeries. It is not recommended in patients with multilocular cysts, infected cysts and cysts with biliary communication. Spillage, anaphylaxis and recurrence are the complications associated with PAIR technique.

Operative Management

It includes either the open surgery or the laparoscopic surgery. The open surgical method will be discussed in this chapter, while the laparoscopic procedure and percutaneous aspiration will be discussed in appropriate section.

All the patients with symptomatic cysts and asymptomatic patients with cyst size more than 4 cm in diameter are candidates for surgery. All infected and ruptured cysts need surgical intervention. If the patient has multiple cysts, only superficial and accessible cysts should be considered for surgery, and the surgery of remaining cysts can be delayed until they become superficial. The cysts smaller than 4 cm, cysts located deep within the liver substance more than 4 cm below the liver capsule and calcified cysts are managed conservatively (Ibrahim 2016). Those with deep cysts should not be operated upon as the surgeon must cut through a thick layer of normal tissue to reach the cyst. In these deep-seated cysts, it is better to follow these patients by six monthly sonographic examinations and should be operated only once they reach to the surface of the liver. On the other hand, most of the calcified cysts have stopped growing and do not pose any threat to the patient. Besides it, the calcified cyst cavity is difficult to close after surgery, and also it does not get obliterated as the wall is stiff and calcareous. If in such patients infection of the cavity occurs, it will result in non-healing abscess formation.

The principles of operative management include preoperative preparation, adequate exposure of the cyst, minimal mobilization of the liver and the cyst to avoid iatrogenic perforation, isolation of the area containing cyst with gauze packs soaked with a protoscolicidal solution, prevention of spillage of cyst contents during surgery, opening and evacuation of hydatid cavity should be carried out in a closed system in modern hydatid surgery both in open method or laparoscopic approach, identification and management of any cysto-biliary communication if any and management of residual cavity.

There are two basic surgical methods for managing hepatic hydatidosis (Malik et al. 2008):

A. Radical operative procedures
B. Conservative surgical procedure

Radical Operative Procedures

Several surgeons particularly from developed countries advocate radical surgical procedures with good results. There are several radical surgical methods for managing the hydatid cyst of the liver. These include pericystectomy also known as cysto-pericystectomy, which could be open cysto-pericystectomy or closed cysto-pericystectomy (Malik et al. 2008), hepatic resection and wedge resection. Since the integrity of the cyst is not breached in these procedures and chances of accidental contamination of peritoneal content are less, therefore there is no need of aspiration of cyst contents and use of scolicidal agents (Zinner et al. 1997). There is considerable blood loss as there is no clear plane of dissection between the pericyst and the hepatic parenchyma. However, in the hands of an experienced person, mortality may be as low as 5%, with these radical procedures.

Closed Total Cysto-pericystectomy It involves en bloc excision of the intact cyst including the pericyst in the plane between the pericyst and liver parenchyma. Some authors have favoured it arguing that the risk of spillage into peritoneal cavity is low, and it leads to more rapid closure of remaining cavity. However, this method involves major liver resection with increase in operative risk, postoperative bleeding and bile leakage. Sometimes, there may be massive bleeding which may be difficult to control. It should be reserved for peripherally placed cysts, pedunculated cysts, extrahepatic intra-abdominal cysts and calcified cysts (Malik et al. 2008). This procedure is contraindicated for cysts which are impinging on the major hepatic veins, inferior vena cava and those close to hilum.

Open Total Cysto-pericystectomy In some patients, while doing the closed total cystopericystectomy, one may inadvertently enter into the cyst or encounter a major hepatic vein or there may be impending rupture. In such cases, closed cystopericystectomy is abandoned and converted into open cysto-pericystectomy. The cyst is decompressed and sterilized in usual manner and remaining pericyst resected from the liver parenchyma.

Hepatic Resection It is indicated if the liver parenchyma of one lobe is destroyed by the huge cyst or there are multiple cysts in one lobe or bilobar cyst is found close to the main vascular structure (Milicevic 2005; Malik et al. 2008). However, it is associated with high morbidity and mortality.

Wedge Resection It is useful for patients with peripherally located, multiloculated cysts.

Postoperative complications are less frequent when complete excision is performed. The incidence of biliary fistula is only 10% with radical procedures as compared to 25% in patients who undergo conservative surgical procedures. Similarly, recurrence rate is also less than 2% in radical procedures as compared to 25% seen with conservative surgical procedures (Milicevic 2005).

Conservative Surgical Method

Cystectomy is the most common conservative surgical method performed worldwide. It is the simplest and safest surgical method and a preferred choice for most of the patients. This involves evacuation of all the contents of the cyst including germinal lining, daughter cysts, hydatid fluid and scoleces, leaving the pericyst behind. This is followed by irrigation of the cavity with a scolicidal agent and management of the residual pericystic cavity (Malik et al. 2008). Hypertonic saline (15%), chlorhexidine (10%), ethanol 80%, hydrogen peroxide 3%, povidone iodine 1%, silver nitrate 0.5% and cetrimide 0.5% have been used as scolicidal agent. These scolicidal agents kill almost 80–90% of scoleces. These scolicidal agents are not able to sterilize multilocular cysts and can lead to inflammation and cholangitis if the cyst has communication with the biliary tract. Scolicidal agents are not used if the aspirate is bile stained or if it is purulent as one should suspect a biliary communication. The scolicidal agent should also not be injected if the cyst is multilocular.

Preoperative Preparation

Antihistamines should be administered preoperatively to the patients, and corticosteroids and epinephrine should be kept available in the event of intraoperative anaphylactic shock. A single dose of antibiotics should be given as a prophylaxis half an hour before surgery.

Incision and Approach

It should be decided before surgery whether to go for an abdominal approach, thoracic approach or a thoracoabdominal approach. It can be arbitrarily decided preoperatively by drawing an imaginary line at the level of the xiphoid. Cysts lying above this imaginary line are better approached through the chest, and those below this are approached through the abdomen. Similarly, if the cyst can be palpated on the abdomen below the costal margin, they are also approached through the abdominal incision, while cysts with intrathoracic rupture are better approached through chest. It is because that the entry into the cyst should be through the most superficial part of the cyst that we should be able to lay open the entire cystic cavity so that the cyst is completely evacuated of its contents; otherwise, there are high chances of persistence of disease, infection and recurrence. The most common approach through the chest is via standard poster lateral incision, usually the eighth or ninth intercostal space.

Most of the hydatid cysts of the liver are approached through abdominal incision. We have been routinely using right subcostal incision in our practice except for patients with intraperitoneal rupture, where a right paramedian or midline incision is made. Some surgeons are comfortable with rooftop incision (bilateral subcostal) which provides excellent access to all cysts except for the cyst located in the most posterior part of the liver. Abdominal incisions allow exploration of the peritoneum for any concurrent cysts and also manual and sonographic evaluation of the entire lobe for any additional cysts. For patients where biliary involvement is suspected, the abdominal approach is the ideal one as it allows proper exposure of biliary system, intraoperative cholangiography and any subsequent procedure if needed. Presence of both the superior but partly intrathoracic cyst and inferior abdominal cyst warrants individual incision, and sometimes even we need to operate at different timings.

Mobilization and Isolation

Once the peritoneal cavity is entered, the abdomen should be thoroughly explored. The liver should be completely mobilized, and any adhesion found between the diaphragm and liver should be carefully separated. Bimanual palpation and inspection of both the lobes are mandatory. If there is a large posterior cyst in the liver that is firmly adherent to the diaphragm, it may be difficult to separate, and it is better to perform separate thoracotomy. Sometimes, it may be difficult to locate the cyst by inspection or palpation; in such cases intraoperative ultrasonography should be carried out to look for the most superficial part of the cyst through which the cyst can be approached.

Decompression

The superficial part of the cyst is easily seen as a distinct area from its colour or consistency, quite different from the rest of the surrounding liver (Fig. 1). Before any further manipulation is done, the area harbouring the cyst is walled off from the rest of the operative area by placing large packs which have been soaked in any of the available scolicidal solutions. The edges of the abdominal or chest incision are also covered by separate packs soaked in scolicidal solution to avoid any contamination by hydatid fluid are any implantation by daughter cysts. The viable hydatid cyst is under high pressure, and the pressure could be as high as 70 cm of water (Kattan et al. 1977), and some degree of leakage of hydatid fluid may occur during surgery. To avoid this, the first step should be to lower the intracystic pressure. Several methods can be used to decompress the cyst.

1. The cyst is decompressed by inserting a large-bore angiocath needle, and the colour of hydatid fluid is observed (Malik et al. 2008). About 50 ml of hydatid fluid is aspirated with a syringe to reduce the cystic pressure. It is important to see the colour of contents to rule out any biliary communication. The contents are bile stained in case there is any biliary communication, and in such cases, injection of scolicidal agents should be avoided. After the decompression has been done, a scolicidal solution is injected into the cavity and left there for 10 min. The quantity of scolicidal agent injected should be less than the aspirated volume of hydatid fluid (Malik et al. 2008). This technique fails if the cyst is multivesicular as only one or two daughter cysts are punctured.

2. The cyst can also be punctured with a suction catheter and is quite effective in both univesicular cyst and multivesicular cyst (Fig. 2).
3. Saidi's Technique: decompression can be done by using a Saidi's cone (Saidi 1977). This instrument consists of a cone; lower end of this cone is placed on the most superficial part of the cyst. The end of the cone remains fastened with the surface of the cyst either by a simple suction attachment or by rapid freezing mechanism incorporated into the circular lower end of the cone.
4. Aarons Technique: decompression can be performed by using another cone devised by Aarons and Kune in 1983. This instrument consists of two concentric cylinders with a separate suction arrangement and a long handled knife at the top of the inside of the inner cylinder. The lower end of the outer cylinder remains attached to the surface of the liver by a simple suction, while the lower end of the inner cylinder sucks out cyst contents after the pericyst is incised by the knife provided with the instrument.

Evacuation of the Cyst Contents

After the cyst is decompressed by any of the methods to lower the cyst pressure, two stay sutures are applied close to the punctured area. The cyst wall is incised between these two stay sutures with the help of electrocautery and a large gauge suction drain inserted and suction continued. The incision is further enlarged in size to several centimetres, so that there is direct vision of the inside of the cavity, and all the cyst contents are removed including the laminated membrane, daughter cyst and debris (Figs. 3, 4, 5, 6, 7, 8 and 9). The cyst is rarely removed intact as it has already ruptured and is usually removed in piecemeal with the help of suction curette (Morris and Lamont 1987). The laminated membrane is best managed by a ring forcep. It is sometimes necessary to use a spoon to evacuate daughter cysts. The removal of cyst contents of a univesicular cyst may be quite simple, but it is tedious to remove the contents of a large multivesicular cyst as there may be large number of small and large daughter cysts along with a jelly-like material.

It is important to see the colour of contents to rule out any biliary communication. In those cases where there is any biliary communication, the contents will be bile stained, and in such cases, injection of scolicidal agents should be avoided. In some cases, the contents are not bile stained, but later on, after evacuation of the contents, biliary communications become apparent. The logic behind is that there exists a valvular mechanism, and these valves open once the intracystic pressure decreases after the contents have been evacuated. That is why at the end of the procedure, cavity is examined for any bile duct communication, which if found has to be closed with vicryl suture (Malik et al. 2008). The pericyst cavity is then opened widely and the overlying ectocyst excised to de-roof the cyst (Fig. 10). The cavity is again examined, and if any contents are found, they are removed. Once all the contents are removed, the cavity is rinsed with 3–5% warm saline. Finally, the cavity is scraped with a gauze soaked in scolicidal solution (Fig. 11). Curettage with sharp instruments is avoided as it can cause damage to the hepatic veins. The cavity is again checked for any bile leakage. The cavity is then packed with white gauze soaked in normal saline and kept there for few minutes. If there is any bile staining of the gauze, the cavity needs to be re-examined, and if any biliary communication is found, that needs to be managed.

After the surgeon is sure that there is no biliary communication, sterilization of the cavity is carried out using any of the available scolicidal agents. The solution should be kept in the cavity for at least 5–10 min, after which the solution should be aspirated. At this stage, we should examine the whole liver for any non-palpable cyst, and if any of them is accessible, they should be also dealt with. Intraoperative ultrasonography is quite a useful diagnostic tool in such cases. On the other hand, small and deep cyst may be left as such. It is always better to palpate the walls of the residual cavity with the fingertips to feel for any additional cysts lying just outside the cavity. These additional cysts can be managed from the inner surface of the already evacuated pericystic cavity.

Fig. 1 Intact hydatid cyst in the right lobe of the liver

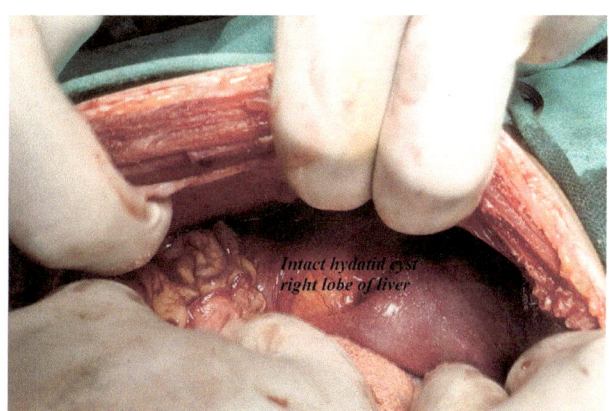

Fig. 2 Hydatid cyst in the right lobe of the liver

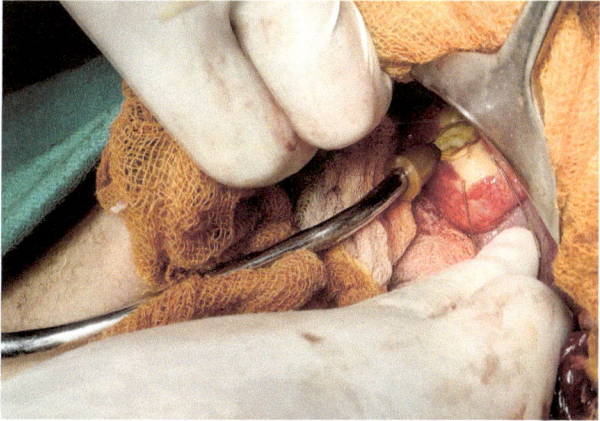

Fig. 3 Laminated
membrane being evacuated
from hydatid cyst cavity

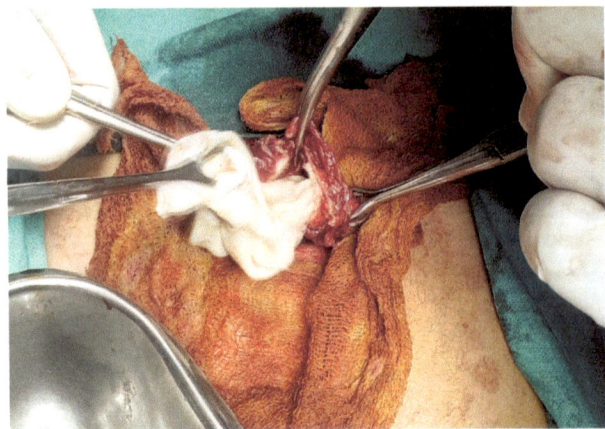

Fig. 4 Ruptured hydatid
cyst in the left lobe of the
liver

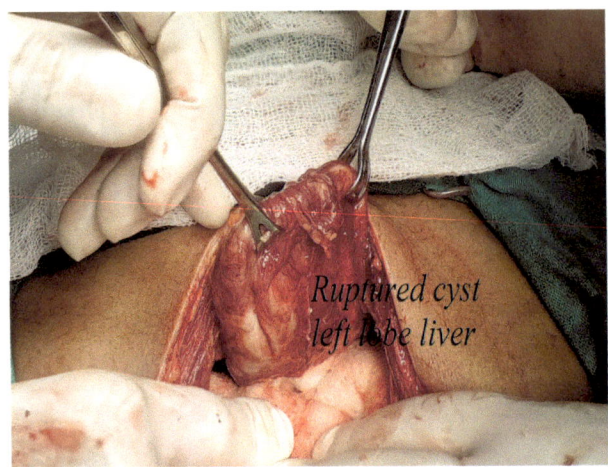

*Ruptured cyst
left lobe liver*

Fig. 5 Laminated
membrane of hydatid cyst

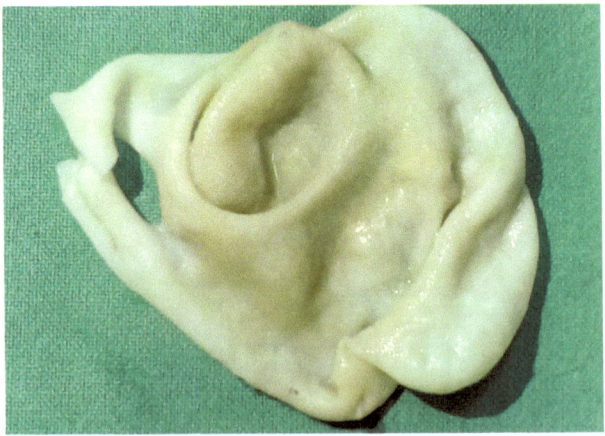

Fig. 6 Bile-stained laminated membrane removed from cyst cavity

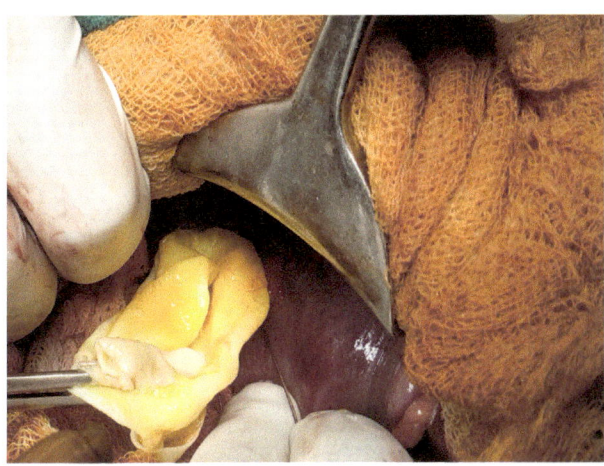

Fig. 7 Operative photograph showing completely evacuated cyst cavity

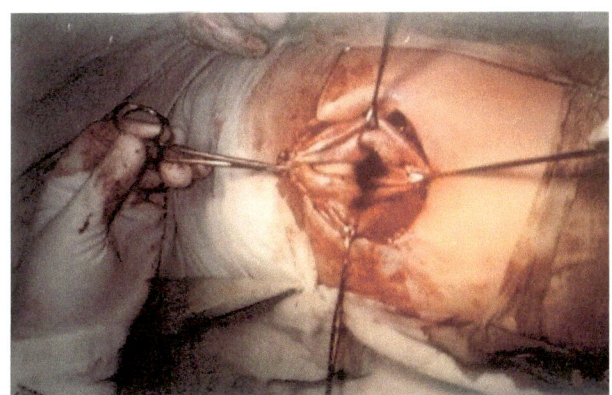

Fig. 8 Multiple daughter cysts removed from the hydatid cyst of the liver

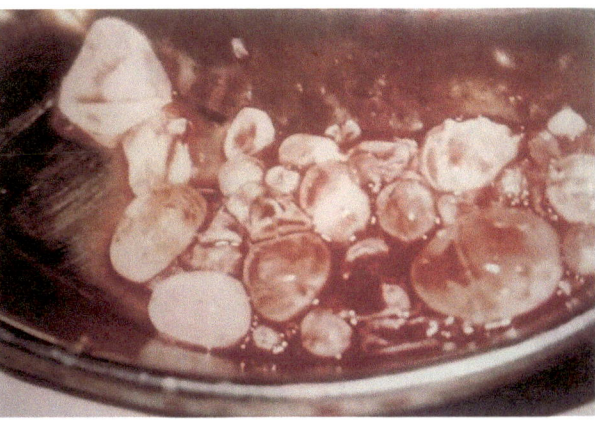

Fig. 9 Large laminated membrane removed from the hydatid cyst of the liver

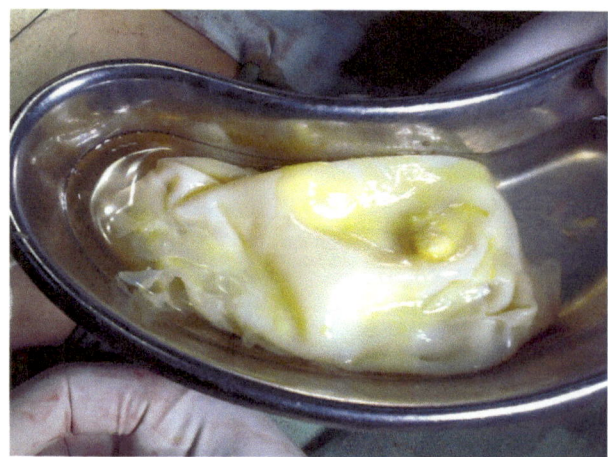

Fig. 10 Pericyst excised after de-roofing of the cyst cavity

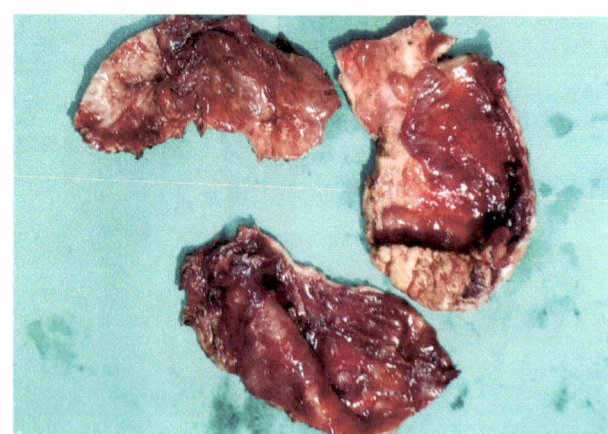

Fig. 11 Rinsing of the cavity being done using gauze soaked in scolicidal agent

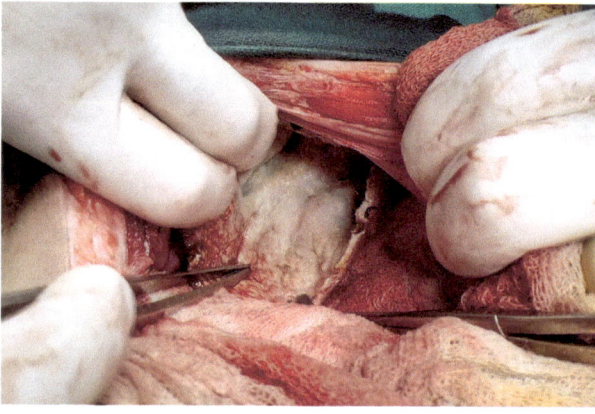

Scolicidal Agents Used in Hydatid Liver Surgery

A number of protoscolicidal agents have been used since decades for sterilizing the cyst. While using any of the available scolicidal agents, several things are to be kept in consideration which include concentration, volume, time of contact and safety of the scolicidal agent. The need for using these scolicidal agents is based on the fact that spillage may occur during surgery or some daughter cysts may get implanted on the surface of pericystic cavity or may get implanted in the surrounding areas resulting in regrowth of new cysts in the future. The best way of killing these unseen scoleces and thereby preventing the recurrence is to fill the cavity with effective scolicidal agent. Although use of scolicidal agents is an essential step in conservative hydatid liver surgery and using a proper scolicidal agent in proper concentration and adequate quantity is mandatory, they cannot be a substitute for a proper meticulous technique. Even the most effective scolicidal may not kill the protoscoleces as these scolicidal agents do not penetrate the wall of daughter cyst. The following scolicidal agents have been used for the last several decades by different surgeons and researchers:

1. *Formalin*: It was the most commonly used scolicidal agent in the past. However, it is no longer used now as it has been found to cause fatal systemic toxicity (Barros 1978; Fraya et al. 1981) and has high propensity to cause sclerosing cholangitis in patients with biliary communications. Formalin should never be injected into any cyst cavity regardless of the size of cyst and the volume to be used and whether the communication is there or not as it is a very strong denaturant for any of the surrounding tissues.
2. *Silver nitrate*: Saidi and Nazarian in 1977 strongly advocated the use of dilute silver nitrate (0.5%) and found excellent clinical results. After that, several authors have used freshly prepared 0.5% silver nitrate to sterilize the cyst cavity. It is a cheap, readily available, nontoxic and effective scolicidal agent. However, it has got a contact period of 10 min and is not safe if there are biliary communications as it can cause caustic sclerosing cholangitis (Frayha et al. 1971).
3. *Hypertonic saline*: Several studies have been carried using different concentrations of hypertonic saline (3–30%). It has been found quite effective against scoleces at a concentration of more than 15%. The higher the concentration, the more the scolicidal activity with shorter contact period. Twenty per cent hypertonic saline has 100% scolicidal activity with contact period of 6 min.
4. *Povidone-iodine* (Polyvinylpyrrolidone-iodine): Povidone-iodine in the concentration of 10% is an effective agent for prevention of secondary hydatidosis. In vitro studies in animals have found it more effective than hypertonic saline in preventing peritoneal infection (Gokce et al. 1991). However, its effect on biliary tree in humans and potential systemic complications due to absorption of iodine are yet not clear. Colouring of cystic cavity is the main disadvantage of this solution making it difficult to identify the cysto-biliary communication.

5. *Cetrimide* (cetyltrimethylammonium bromide): Cetrimide is an effective scolicidal agent and has been used for sterilizing the cyst cavities since 1978 (Ahrari et al. 1978). Since it is a potent and toxic agent, it should be used in low concentrations of 0.1%, 0.5% and 1%. However, its use has been found to be associated with chemical peritonitis and massive adhesions (Gilchrist 1979). Other problems with cetrimide include metabolic acidosis and caustic sclerosing cholangitis.

6. *Cetrimide and chlorhexidine*: Combination of both cetrimide 0.5% and chlorhexidine 0.05% with contact period of 5 min is an effective protoscolicidal agent. Side effects such as metabolic acidosis and methaemoglobinaemia are reported in the literature.

7. *Absolute alcohol*: It is effective in higher concentrations of 75–95% but is not used in patients with biliary communication or those with a communication with peritoneal cavity (Filice et al. 1990). It is used mostly for sclerosis and is not effective on protoscoleces inside daughter cysts. Caustic cholangitis and being highly flammable are other disadvantages.

8. *Hydrogen peroxide*: Hydrogen peroxide has also been used as a scolicidal agent in the concentration of 1.5–3%. However, it is more effective when used in a concentration of more than 10%, but at this concentration, it can cause lethal air embolism and anaphylactic shock. Another drawback of hydrogen peroxide is that bursting of the cyst with spillage of cyst contents can occur when hydrogen peroxide is injected into the cyst (Belghiti et al. 1986; Djilall et al. 1983).

Word About Sclerosing Cholangitis

This is an extremely serious condition and a late complication reported by several authors in those patients who have underwent hydatid cyst surgery, and surgeons have used any of the available scolicidal agents whether it be formalin, ethanol, silver nitrate, cetrimide or hypertonic saline (Belghiti et al. 1986; Teres et al. 1984). The relative risk of different scolicidal agents has not been determined yet. The cysto-biliary communication may be seen in as many as 5–30% cases, and improper use of such toxic agents may result into caustic damage of the biliary tree, leading to sclerosing cholangitis. It is because of this that most of the authors do not recommend injection of scolicidal agent into the unopened cyst. Rather the contents should be removed and the cavity cleaned meticulously and searched for any biliary communication before using any of the available scolicidal agents. This sclerosing cholangitis is a life-threatening condition and should be suspected in any patient who has underwent hydatid liver surgery with or without proved cysto-biliary communication and where scolicidal agents have been used intraoperatively.

Management of Residual Cavity

The method for managing the residual cavity after evacuation of contents must be selected carefully. Simple cyst closure, marsupialization, leaving the cyst cavity open, captionage, omentoplasty, introflexion external tube drainage, Roux-en-Y cystojejunostomy and hepatic resection are the various options available depending on size, site and number of cyst and the preference of the surgeon. Primary obliteration of the cyst cavity using omentum or captionage has been used successfully and has shown better results (Malik et al. 2008; Sheikh et al. 2001), but cysts need to be uncomplicated. The various techniques that have been used to manage the residual cavity are:

1. *Marsupialization*: Initially, the residual cyst cavities were dealt with by marsupialization (Wani et al. 2005; Malik et al. 2008). In this, the edges of the opening of the pericyst cavity are sutured to the skin, thereby allowing free drainage of the cavity to the exterior. This procedure is ideal for infected cysts, but it invariably results into a large open infected skin wound draining the bile, which may persist for several months and may be difficult to close. In some cases, haemorrhage can occur. In view of unacceptably high rates of complications (Papadimitrio and Mandrakes 1970), this procedure fell into disregard.

2. *Open drainage*: Wide open drainage of the cyst cavity into the peritoneal cavity is practiced in case of small, superficial and large shallow uninfected cysts which may be otherwise difficult to close. The edge of the cavity is overrun with catgut sutures but otherwise left open. There are some prerequisites for doing such a procedure. One is that the cavity should be univesicular and second is that the cavity has to be shallow so that the loops of the intestine do not get entrapped in it.

3. *Saline-tight closure/capsulorrhaphy*: In this, the opening of the pericyst cavity is sutured watertight using running absorbable sutures without any drain. The cavity is then filled with a sterile saline or can be even left open. This method is recommended in patients with small, noncalcified non-infected cysts and univesicular cyst with no major biliary communication. Fluid which is left in the cavity will drain off through existing small bile duct openings. There is a small risk of secondary infection of the fluid, which may sometimes necessitate second procedure either open or under sonographic guidance.

4. *Captionage*: Here the dead space is obliterated by a series of purse string sutures starting from bottom of the pericyst towards the surface. This method is an alternative to omentopexy, if enough omentum is not available. While applying sutures, one has to be very careful to avoid deep sutures; otherwise, injury to hepatic veins can occur. However, this method cannot be used when the cavity is too large and the cyst wall is calcified and rigid.

5. *Omentopexy*: Here a viable flap of omentum is brought to rest within the pericyst cavity with the assumption that omentum will seal small biliary leaks and obliterate the cavity as well (Malik et al. 2008). This method was described by Papadimitrion and Mandrekas in 1970 and is considered as a management of choice for dealing with residual hepatic hydatid cyst cavity as it is associated with less morbidity, short hospital stay and less recurrence as compared to external tube drainage. This method is particularly recommended for patients with a deep cyst cavity in the posterior part of the liver. In patients with a large cavity, this method can be combined with an external tube drainage (Malik et al. 2008).

6. *Introflexion*: It is a modification of captionage in which the upper edge of the pericyst is rolled in and is sutured to the deepest part of cavity with absorbable sutures and then the other edge of the pericyst is sutured to collapsed edge by a running suture.

7. *External tube drainage*: In this an appropriate diameter tube drain is placed in the cyst cavity and brought out through a separate opening. This procedure is used in patients with infected cyst and cysts with biliary communication. The tube drain is placed in the cavity till no fluid drains out during last 48 h or till the time cavity obliterates. Obliteration of the cavity is confirmed by performing sonogram biweekly, and the tube is pulled out once the cavity has shrunken to a small track. During our study on an average, the tube had to be placed for 5–6 days in case of simple cysts and for 10–14 days in case of complicated cysts. It is a treatment of choice for patients with infected hydatid cyst. Although there were initial reports of successful treatment by enucleation and external tube drainage, problems of increased infection and prolonged drainage and fistulae were noted (Malik et al. 2010).

8. *Hepatic resection*: Liver resection is usually not done as it seems to be too radical for managing a benign condition.

Management of Bile Duct Communications

A special problem arises when there is an intrabiliary rupture of hydatid cysts of the liver (Alper 1987). In such cases, it is essential to identify the communication and manage the cyst as well as biliary communication in one sitting. Intrabiliary communication should always be suspected in patients with large cysts more than 10 cm, cyst involving several segments of the liver and inferior vena cava invasion, degenerative cyst and larger surface area of hepatectomy and in patients where the USG shows hydatid debris in bile ducts, with history of biliary colic, with history of cholangitis and where the preoperative endoscopic retrograde cholangiography (ERCP) has demonstrated the presence of membranes and cyst in the biliary tract. Several multivariate analyses have also shown that there are several biochemical parameters that predict a biliary communication which include total serum bilirubin level of more than 0.8 mg/dl, alanine aminotransferase (ALT) > 28U/L, ALP > 165 U/L, lactate dehydrogenase (LDH) > 194 U/L and blood loss > 450 mL. In such patients where there is a biliary communication, contents are bile stained. Demircan et al. reported that high levels of direct bilirubin, ALP and LDH were independent risk factors of biliary leakage. The liver is one of the major organs that produce LDH which is released into the peripheral blood following liver cell death caused by ischaemia or injury. High LDH levels may also reflect the number of affected bile ducts and the severity of liver injury.

However absence of bile staining does not rule out biliary communication. Intraoperative cholangiography should be done to demonstrate the presence of biliary communication, although it will not localize the site of leak. Several other methods have been used to confirm the leak. One method is to take a white gauze soaked in saline solution, place it in the cavity and wait for a few minutes. The gall bladder is then compressed gently, and white gauze is examined. In patients with a biliary communication, the gauze will be bile stained. After this, the cavity is thoroughly searched for the biliary communications. The other methods are to fill the cavity with a saline, inject air and look for air bubbles at the site of biliary leak. Some authors inject methylene blue into the gall bladder or CBD, but the disadvantage of this method is that everything is stained blue and it may be difficult to localize the communication (Milicevic 2005).

Once the biliary communication is identified, the fibrous tissue lying over the bile duct is cleared. The direction of the bile duct is determined by gentle probing of the duct using a thin curved probe (Ibrahim 2016). Some authors use a soft plastic cannula to cannulate duct, inject a dye and perform fluorocholangiography to demonstrate the biliary tree. Presence of any membranes or daughter cyst in the biliary tree can be seen with the help of fluorocholangiography. Further management depends on the calibre of the duct involved, location of the communication and the status of common bile duct (Alper 1987).

In patients with a small peripheral duct involvement, simple suture using vicryl is all what is to be done. This procedure is needed in most of the patients with bile-stained contents. When a larger bile duct is involved or hydatid debris is found in the CBD, exploration of CBD should be done via supraduodenal choledochotomy, all the debris should be removed and T-tube should be placed along with tension-free closure of peripheral communication. In some patients, the cyst may be close to the hilum of the liver and may be communicating with a major duct. In such cases, if closure of such communications is attempted, it may compromise the biliary drainage. The ideal procedure in these cases is to bring a Roux-en-loop of the jejunum close to the superficial part of the cyst and anastomose it with the cyst wall – procedure known as Roux-en-Y cystojejunostomy. In some cases with markedly dilated CBD filled with debris, with major duct disruption, T-tube drainage is combined with Roux-en-Y cystojejunostomy. In some cases with major duct disruption within the cyst, intracystic Roux-en-Y hepaticojejunostomy is done. In these patients, the jejunum is directly sutured to the duct opening within the cyst cavity. Roux-en-Y hepaticojejunostomy is also performed in those patients where the confluence is damaged or destroyed.

In patients whose CBD is markedly dilated and is filled with daughter cysts, hydatid debris and membranes, choledochoduodenostomy may be performed, although many authors prefer Roux-en-Y hepaticojejunostomy (Milicevic 2005) in these patients as well. In patients with obstructed papilla by calcified debris or any other reason, sphincteroplasty may be done either by open or endoscopic method (Zargar et al. 1992).

Liver resection is an uncommon method of managing biliary communication and is done in patients with atrophic and fibrotic liver with compromised liver functions but is accompanied with serious complications.

Complications of Surgery

Several complications are encountered in the postoperative period in patients undergoing hydatid liver surgery. The early postoperative complications are bile leakage, liver abscess, subphrenic abscess and the wound infection, while recurrence is a late complication.

Bile Leakage Biliary leakage as proposed by the International Study Group of Liver Surgery (ISGLS) is defined as a drainage of fluid with a bilirubin level three times greater than the serum level on or after third postoperative day or the need for interventions because of bile collection or biliary peritonitis. Biliary leak that requires no or little change in a clinical management of the patient is considered as Grade A leakage, while biliary leaks that require additional diagnostic or interventional procedures are considered as Grade B leakage. Grade A leakage which lasts for more than 1 week is also classified as Grade B leakage, while bile leak which requires re-exploration is considered as Grade C leakage.

Bile leakage is a relatively common but a self-limiting problem. A biliary fistula should be suspected if there is a drainage of large quantity of bile in the early postoperative period. It could be due to an overlooked cysto-biliary communication or inadequately managed cysto-biliary communication, obstruction of the distal bile duct by hydatid membranes or daughter cysts or iatrogenic injury to bile duct. Whatever the reason, early management should be conservative .The tube drain should be retained for 2–3 weeks as most of the bile leaks close within this period of time. In some cases, it will be worthwhile to wait for a few more weeks. In our clinical practice, we have retained the tube for as many as 6 weeks (Malik et al. 2010). If biliary fistula continues or it is a high out fistula (>300 ml), the patient will need an ERCP along with papillotomy. In most of the cases, there is no need to place a stent, and the success rate is from 90 to 100%. Patients with prolonged bile leak may need re-operation for localization and suturing of cysto-biliary fistula. Some patients may need biliary decompression procedures such as T-tube drainage, transduodenal sphincterotomy and choledochoduodenostomy or may need internal drainage such as cystojejunostomy.

Liver Abscess It is a less common complication as usually de-roofing of the cavity is done, although some authors have reported it up to the extent of 8% (Milicevic 2005). If it occurs, pus can be drained percutaneously under ultrasound guidance. Open drainage of pus is rarely needed.

Mortality Mortality in hydatid disease could be due to an anaphylactic shock following traumatic rupture and hepatic failure due to cirrhosis. In the past, intraoperative formalin toxicity was one of the causes for mortality in these patients. However, formalin is no longer used now. The overall mortality rates vary from one series to another. Papadimitrio and Mandrakes (1970) reported a hospital mortality of 3.5%, and Christopher and Lopez (1970) reported mortality of 9%, while there was no mortality in a series reported by Belli et al. (1983).

Recurrence Recurrence is one of the major complications of hydatid surgery and usually occurs several years after initial surgery. Recurrence can be local, regional or distant. Different authors have defined recurrence in different ways. Some authors define recurrence as a growing cyst at the site of initial operative (Amir-Jehad et al. 1975), while others define it as appearance of cyst at the new site (Little et al. 1988). The incidence of recurrence has been reported variably as it is not well established, and it depends on the length and quality of follow-up. Long-term postoperative follow-up is needed to establish the recurrence. Ultrasound of the abdomen is the simplest and a reliable non-invasive investigation to follow these patients, which should be repeated every 6 months. Computed tomography and MRI may be needed only in those patients where there is any doubt in diagnosis. The recurrence is more in conservative surgery as compared to radical surgery (Zinner et al. 1997). Amir-Jehad et al. (1975) have reported a recurrence rate of only 0.9%, while recurrence rate has been reported as 2.2% by Gilevich et al. (1980), 5% by Little (1976), 8.5% by Barros, 11.3% by Mottaghion and Saidi (1978) and 22% by Little et al. (1988).

It is important to understand that the cause of recurrence is the spillage of hydatid fluid and implantation of daughter cysts during initial surgery and the chances of spillage are more in a viable cyst filled with active daughter cysts. The likelihood of recurrence is also more in patients where there has been a spontaneous rupture of the cyst with the seeding of daughter cysts in the peritoneal cavity. Rate of recurrence is substantially reduced by preventing spillage during initial surgery and prophylactic use of albendazole therapy both before surgery and after surgery (Bari et al. 2011). The management of recurrence of hydatid cyst depends on the choice of surgeon. Many authors have managed recurrence with chemotherapy only as the second surgery is quite tedious. There are lots of adhesions, dissection may be difficult, there will be considerable blood loss, and there are chances of iatrogenic injury. However, some patients may need a second surgery to control the disease.

References

Ahrari H. Use of cetrimide in the surgery of hydatid cyst. Bull Soc Pathol Exot Filiales. 1978;71:90–4.
Alper A. Choledochoduodenostomy for intrabiliary rupture of hydatid cysts of liver. Br J Surg. 1987;74(4):243–5.
Amir-Jehad AK, Faria R, Furzad R. Clinical echinococcus. Ann Surg. 1975;182:541–5.
Arif SH, Bari S u, Wani NA, Zargar SA. Albendazole as an adjuvant to the standard surgical management of hydatid cyst liver. Int J Surg. 2008;6:448–51.
Bari S, S H, Malik AA, Rouf KA, Tufale AD, Zahoor AN. Role of albendazole in the management of hydatid cyst liver. Saudi J Gastroenterol. 2011;17(5):343–7.
Barros JL. Hydatid disease in liver. Am J Surg. 1978;135:597–600.
Belghiti J, Benhamou JP, Pernicerit T. Caustic sclerosing cholangitis: a complication of surgical treatment of hydatid disease of the liver. Arch Surg. 1986;121:1162–5.
Belli L, del Favero E, Marni A. Resection versus pericystectomy in the treatment of hydatidosis of the liver. Am J Surg. 1983;145(2):239–42.
Christopher PJ, Lopez WA. Hydatid disease notifications in New South Wales. Med J Aust. 1970;1:1773–5.
Djilall G, Mehrour A, Cussedlk T. L'eau oxygenee dans la chirurgie du Kyste hydatique. La Presse Medicale. 1983;12:235–7.
Filice C, Pirola F, Brunetti E. A new therapeutic approach for hydatid cyst. Aspiration and alcohol injections under sonographic guidance. Gastroenterology. 1990;98:1366–8.
Fraya GJ, Bikhazi KJ, Kachachi TA. Treatment of hydatid cysts (*Echinococcus granulosus*) by cetrimide. Trans R Soc Trop Med Hyg. 1981;75:447–50.
Frayha GJ, Saheb SE, Dajani RM. Systematic research for a systemic scolicide. Chemotherapy. 1971;16:371–9.

Gilchrist DS. Chemical peritonitis after cetrimide washout in hydatid cyst surgery. Lancet. 1979;ii:1374.

Gilevich IS, Ataev BA, Vafin AZ. Relapses in Echinococcus disease (Russ). Vestnik Khirugie. 1980;124:39–45.

Gokce O, Gokce C, Yilmaz M, Huseyinoglu K, Gunel S. Povidone–iodine in experimental peritoneal hydatidosis. Br J Surg. 1991;78:495–6.

Heath DD, Christie MJ, Chevis RAF. The lethal effect of mebendazole on secondary Echinocccos granulosus, cysticerci of Taenia pisiformis and tetrathyridia of mesocestoides corti. Parasitology. 1975;70:273–85.

Ibrahim HH. Hepatic hydatid cysts: management and outcome of open surgical treatment. Eur Surg. 2016;48:290–5.

Kattan YB. Intrabiliary rupture of hydatid cysts of the liver. Ann R Coll Surg Engl. 1977;59:109–14.

Khuroo MS. Hydatid disease: current status and recent advances. Ann Saudi Med. 2002;22:56–64.

Little JM. Hydatid diseases at the Royal Prince Alfred. Hospital 1964–1974. Med J Aust. 1976;1:903–8.

Little JM, Hollands MT, Eckberg H. Recurrence of hydatid disease. World J Surg. 1988;12:700–4.

Malik AA, Bari S, Shah K, Shah FA, Amin R, Jan M. External tube drainage versus omentopexy in the management of residual hepatic hydatid cyst cavity. Int J Surg. 2008;15(1):10–20.

Malik AA, Bari SUL, Amin R, Jan M. Surgical management of complicated hydatid cysts of the liver. World J Gastrointest Surg. 2010;2(2):78.

Milicevic MN. Hydatid disease. In: Blumgart LH, Fong Y, editors. Surgery of the liver and biliary tract, vol. 2. China: WB Saunders; 2005. p. 1167–97.

Morris DL, Lamont G. Suction curette in the management of hydatid cysts. Br J Surg. 1987;74(4):323.

Mottaghion H, Saidi F. Postoperative recurrence of hydatid disease. Br J Surg. 1978;65:237–42.

Papadimitrio J, Mandrakes A. Surgical treatment of hydatid cyst of liver. Br J Surg. 1970;57:431–9.

Saidi F. A new approach to the surgical treatment of hydatid cyst. Ann R Coll Surg Engl. 1977;59:115–20.

Sheikh KA, Wani AA, Nehvi TH, Bari S. Open method versus capitonnage in management of hydatid cyst. Paediatr Surg Int. 2001;17:382–285.

Teres J, Gomez-Moli J, Bruquera M. Sclerosing cholangitis after surgical treatment of hepatic echinococcal cysts. Report on three cases. Am J Surg. 1984;148:694–7.

Wani RA, Malik AA, Chowdri NA, Wani KA, Naqash SH. Primary extrahepatic abdominal hydatidosis. Int J Surg. 2005;3:125–7.

Zargar SA, Khuroo MS, Khan BA, Dar MY. Intrabiliary rupture of hydatid cyst: sonographic and cholangiographic appearances. Gastrointest Radiol. 1992;17:41–4.

Zinner MJ, Schuxirtz SI, Ellis H. Liver abscess and hydatid disease. Maingot's abdominal operations, vol. II. 10th ed. Stamford, CT: Apleton and Lange; 1997. p. 1513–44.

Drug Therapy in Hydatid Disease of the Liver

Medical management of hydatidosis has been tried with many drugs including anti-mony, arsenic, iodides and mercury (Milicevic 2000; Arif et al. 2008). However there was no evidence of any success. Lately the benzimidazole carbamate group of drugs was introduced and was found effective against larval stage of both *E. granulosus* and *E. multilocularis*. This benzimidazole carbamate group of drugs blocks the uptake of glucose in the parasite, thereby causing depletion of its glycogen stores (Arif et al. 2008). The drug causes death of germinal membrane cells, and the cyst loses its ability to maintain haemostasis and integrity (Heath et al. 1975).

Among the benzimidazole group of drugs, mebendazole was the first drug to be used for hydatid disease (Bekhti et al. 1977; Braithwaite 1981). They treated four patients with a dose of 400–600 mg three times a day. The drug was given in 3-week courses for several months. The compound is poorly absorbed, and only less than 10% of orally administered drug is absorbed. The absorption of mebendazole is increased when taken with a fatty meal. The ideal dosage of mebendazole for hyda-tid disease should be 40–60 mg/kg body weight (50 mg/kg at least). However the results of mebendazole therapy in hydatid disease have been reported as less satis-factory (Schantz et al. 1982; Braithwaite et al. 1982). Later on albendazole was introduced with better absorption properties (Morris et al. 1985; El-Mufti 1989). The principal metabolites are albendazole sulphoxide, sulphone and two amino sul-phones. When albendazole is used preoperatively in dose of 10 mg/kg/day for 1 month, most of the protoscoleces get killed, thereby sterilizing hydatid cyst. However, higher effectiveness of albendazole therapy has been reported after 3 months of uninterrupted treatment (Horton 1989; Arif et al. 2008). The plasma and the cyst concentrations of albendazole are 15–40 times higher than those achieved by mebendazole. The fatty meal has been found to increase the absorption of alben-dazole. The usual dosage scheme for albendazole therapy suggested by Horton (1989) is three 28-day courses of 10 mg/kg/day in divided doses separated by 2-week intervals. The same was later endorsed by the WHO (Arif et al. 2008).

Praziquantel is another drug used against hydatid cyst disease of the liver, in the dose of 40–60 mg/kg/day in divided doses. It is the most active and rapid scolicidal

© Springer Nature Singapore Pte Ltd. 2019
A. A. Malik, S. Bari, *Human Abdominal Hydatidosis*,
https://doi.org/10.1007/978-981-13-2152-8_5

agent and is highly effective against protoscoleces (Arif et al. 2008). It is probably the ideal agent for prophylaxis in the preoperative and postoperative setting to prevent implantation of protoscoleces and subsequent recurrences. It is unlikely to be as effective as albendazole in treating whole cyst as it is less active against germinal layer of the hydatid cyst (Arif et al. 2008). It has been shown to be more effective in combination with albendazole than when used alone (Taylor et al. 1988).

Indications of Chemotherapy in Hydatid Disease

Overall evidence shows that chemotherapy may be effective in 30–40% patients with *E. granulosus* infestation. It is most effective for pulmonary hydatid, less effective in liver infestations and ineffective for hydatid disease of the bone, brain and eyes (Taylor et al. 1989). Chemotherapy is effective in small cysts less than 4 cm in diameter, cyst with thin walls and in younger patients (Arif et al. 2008). Larger cysts with an intact laminated membrane and those with the capability of endogenous vesiculation are more resistant to chemotherapy (Taylor et al. 1988). Chemotherapy is probably the only therapy available for *E. multilocularis* and has been found to prolong survival in such patients (Taylor et al. 1988). Among various drugs available, praziquantel is the most effective protoscolicidal agent in *Echinococcus multilocularis*. There are well-established indications of hydatid disease of the liver where drugs can be used.

Drug Therapy as a Primary Medical Therapy

1. Patients who are unfit for surgery either because of age or who are high-risk cases for surgery because of multiple co-morbid conditions.
2. Recurrent disease: Surgery for recurrent hydatid disease is associated with higher morbidity and mortality (Amir-Jehad et al. 1975; Sherlock 1981).
3. Disseminated disease or inoperable disease: Patients with multiple peritoneal cysts, patients with cysts in multiple organs and patients with honeycombed liver due to hundreds of cysts is an indication for chemotherapy. Similarly, in patients with hydatid disease of the vertebral column (bone) which may be unresectable and patients with hydatid disease of pelvic and long bone which may require a mutilating surgery, chemotherapy is a viable option.

Drug Therapy as an Adjuvant Therapy
Drug therapy is mostly used as an adjuvant to surgical intervention because poor results have been obtained when drugs are used alone. It is used both preoperatively and postoperatively.

1. Postoperatively it is indicated in patients, to prevent secondary echinococcosis after spillage during surgery. The treatment should be started immediately and continued for at least 1 month.
2. Preoperative therapy should be given for at least 1 month before surgery. The possible advantages of preoperative chemotherapy for hydatid disease of the liver include:

(a) It decreases the viability of protoscoleces and causes sterilization of the cyst, thus reduces chances of recurrence.

(b) Cysts become flaccid and subsequent surgery becomes easier.

(c) Risk of anaphylaxis is reduced, making surgery safe.

3. Drug therapy is also used as an adjuvant treatment for known residual disease, for example, spinal disease after decompression, where complete excision was not possible, and in such cases, treatment should be at least for 3 months.

4. It has also been widely used as a concomitant therapy with percutaneous drainage (Khuroo 2002).

Recommended Treatment Plan for Albendazole Therapy

The usual dosage scheme for albendazole was suggested by Horton (1989) and later endorsed by the WHO. In this regimen, three 28-day courses of albendazole are given in dose of 10 mg/kg/day in two divided doses separated by 2-week intervals both preoperatively and postoperatively (El-Mufti 1993; Milicevic 2000). Hydatid cyst in the bone and brain may need a prolonged treatment. Before starting treatment, it is important to exclude pregnancy as albendazole has a teratogenic effect. Baseline white blood cell count and liver function test should be done, which should be repeated every 2 weeks to establish hepatotoxicity at the earliest. If the liver function test gets deranged markedly, the drug should be stopped, although mild hepatocellular dysfunction may be expected in patients on albendazole therapy. USG monitoring and serology may also be used during treatment with chemotherapy as follow-up investigation has been described in the next section.

Side Effects of Chemotherapy

Cyst pain, allergic reactions and reversible neutropenia or leukopenia are the common side effects reported in the literature. Some authors have reported glomerulonephritis (French 1984) and agranulocytosis (Wilson and Rausch 1980). Albendazole is potentially teratogenic and embryo toxic; hence, pregnancy should be excluded before starting treatment with albendazole. Reversible hepatocellular dysfunction is frequent in these patients; that is why liver function test should be monitored biweekly in these patients, and if severe derangement of liver functions is seen, drug should be stopped immediately and started only after the liver functions have returned to normal (Morris 1987; Morris and Taylor 1988).

Clinical Studies

A prospective study was undertaken by the authors to assess the utility of albendazole as adjuvant therapy to the standard surgical management of hydatid disease of the liver (Arif et al. 2008; Bari et al. 2011). In this study, albendazole was used in the dose of 10 mg/kg in divided doses as an add-on therapy to surgery, and improved results were seen in 48 patients out of 64, which were statistically significant. Patients were divided into three groups of 16 patients each. In one group, albendazole was given only preoperatively, and in the second group, albendazole was given only postoperatively, while in the third group, it was given both preoperatively and postoperatively. Among those patients who were put on albendazole therapy preoperatively for 2 months, viable cysts were seen in only 9.37% patients at the time of surgery. On the other hand, viable cysts were seen in 96.87% of patients who did not receive any preoperative albendazole therapy. This decrease in viability of cysts was found to be statistically significant ($p < 0.01$) and indicates that 2 months of preoperative course of albendazole kills most of protoscoleces within hydatid cysts (Arif et al. 2008).

These observations are in agreement with some previous studies. In a study conducted by Morris et al. (1987), 16 patients were put on preoperative albendazole therapy in the dose of 10 mg/kg/day for a period of 1 week to 1 month. Fourteen patients were put on albendazole therapy for 1 month, and out of these 14 patients, only 1 patient had viable protoscoleces (Arif et al. 2008). On the other hand, viable protoscoleces were seen at the time of operation in the remaining two patients who received therapy for only 1 and 3 weeks (Morris et al. 1987)

In our study among the patients who received preoperative albendazole, viable cysts were seen in only three patients on microscopic examination, and in all these three patients, multiple daughter cysts were residing inside the mother cyst (Arif et al. 2008). Although protoscoleces in the main cyst were dead, they were still alive in daughter cysts. Our observation was that although preoperative albendazole is successful in eliminating the parasites inside the mother cyst, it is not so effective in killing the scoleces inside the daughter cysts. This is believed to be because of poor penetration of the drug into the daughter cysts residing inside the mother cyst. In a study conducted by Horton (1989), 500 patients were put on 800 mg of albendazole daily in cycles of 28 days with a drug-free interval of 14 days between the cycles. The mean duration of the cycle was 2.5. Out of 500 patients, only 253 patients were evaluated to study the efficacy of albendazole therapy. Surgery was carried out in only 47 patients and out of the them viable cysts were demonstrated in only five (10.6%) patients.

In our study during a follow-up period of 5–6 years, we did not see any recurrence in any of the 16 patients managed with both preoperative and postoperative albendazole (Arif et al. 2008). On the other hand, during the same follow-up period, recurrence rate of 18.75% was observed in the patients who did not receive any albendazole, while there was a recurrence of 4–16% in patients who received either preoperative or postoperative albendazole therapy. Our results were in agreement with the observations made by Evangelos et al. (1995). In their study, 67 patients were evaluated to see the effect of albendazole therapy on recurrence. Eighteen patients were put on mebendazole in the dose of 40 mg/kg/day, and 49 patients were put on albendazole in the dose of 10 mg/kg/day for 5 days before surgery. All those patients who had viable protoscoleces at the time of surgery were put on the same drug for a period of 1 month. There was no recurrence of disease after a follow-up of 15–67 months (average 41 months) in any of the patients. In another study conducted by Mottaghion and Saidi (1978) on 106 patients, a recurrence of 11.3% was observed over a follow-up period of 6 months to 3 years. A recurrence of 22% has been reported by Little et al. (1988) in their study, while no recurrence was reported by Morris (1989) in patients treated with preoperative albendazole for 1 month with a median postoperative follow-up of 28 months (Arif et al. 2008).

Albendazole in dose of 10 mg/kg/day in two equally divided doses is usually well tolerated by the patients. We did not see any severe side effects during our study. Nausea, vomiting and mild abdominal pain were observed in 4% with reversible alopecia in another 4% patients. Leukopenia was seen in one and mild anaemia in one patient put on albendazole therapy. Deranged liver function tests were observed in 16% of patients after albendazole therapy which returned to normal levels within a month after stopping drug. These observations are in agreement with the study conducted by Morris and Taylor (1988) and Horton (1989).

Assessment of the Results of Albendazole Therapy

Results from various studies have concluded that preoperative use of albendazole significantly reduces the viability of cysts at the time of surgery (Osborne 1980; Okelo 1986; Arif et al. 2008). This can be assessed by observing the motility of the scoleces and their ability to exclude 5% eosin (Figs. 1, 2 and 3) under immediate microscopy (Bari et al. 2011). Certain radiographic changes during chemotherapy may indicate the death of a parasite. Some have described the shrinkage of cyst as an indicator of response, while others believe that the increasing density of the cyst contents indicates good response (Morris et al. 1984). Calcification during therapy is regarded by some as the evidence of response (Saimot et al. 1983). There is presently little information relating the effect of albendazole therapy on the serology in patients with hydatid cyst. The level of circulating antigen and IgM circulating immune complexes increases during albendazole therapy followed by rapid fall (Morris and Gould 1982).

Fig. 1 High-power photomicrograph of the cyst aspirate showing multiple viable protoscoleces (no uptake of 5%)

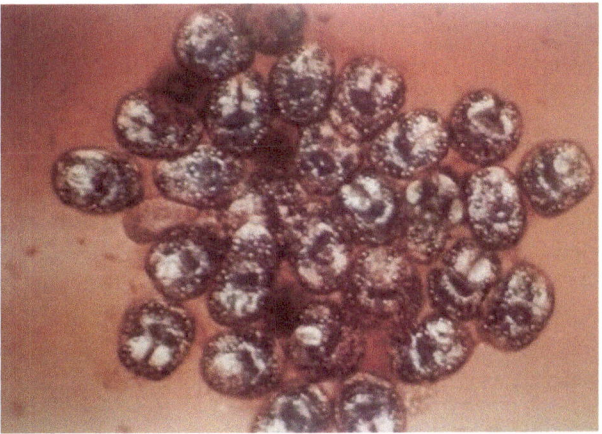

Fig. 2 Photomicrograph
(high power) of cyst
aspirate showing live
protoscolex (able to
exclude 5% eosin)

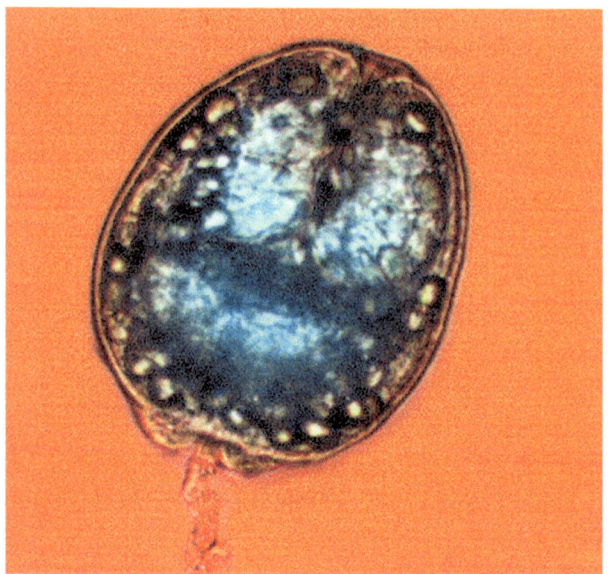

Fig. 3 Photomicrograph
(high power) of cyst
aspirate showing dead
protoscolex – stained with
5% eosin

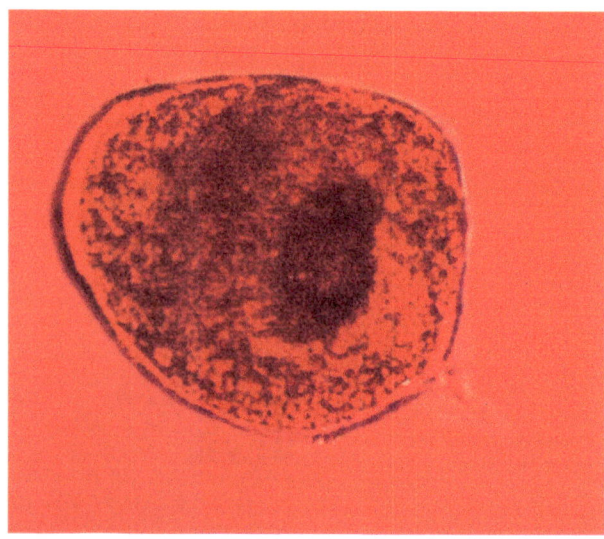

Albendazole therapy is now considered as safe and effective adjuvant therapy in
the management of hepatic hydatid disease in addition to surgery (Arif et al. 2008).
Preoperative use of albendazole significantly decreases the chances of cyst viability
at the time of surgery, while postoperative use of albendazole also decreases the
chances of cyst recurrence (Arif et al. 2008). When albendazole is used both preoperatively and postoperatively, it reduces the chances of the preoperative cyst viability as well as the postoperative cyst recurrence.

References

Amir-Jehad AK, Faria R, Furzad R. Clinical echinococcus. Ann Surg. 1975;182:541–5.

Arif SH, bari S u, Wani NA, Zargar SA. Albendazole as an adjuvant to the standard surgical management of hydatid cyst liver. Int J Surg. 2008;6(6):448–51.

Bari S, S H, Malik AA, Rouf KA, Tufale AD, Zahoor AN. Role of albendazole in the management of hydatid cyst liver. Saudi J Gastroenterol. 2011;17(5):343–7.

Bekhti A, Schaaps JP, Capron M, Dessaint JP, Santoro F, Capron A. Treatment of hepatic hydatid disease with mebendazole: preliminary results in four cases. Br Med J. 1977;ii:1047–51.

Braithwaite PA. Long term high dose mebendazole for cystic disease of liver: failure in two cases. Aust N Z J Surg. 1981;51:23–7.

Braithwaite PA, Roberts MS, Allan RJ. Clinical pharmacokinetics of high dose of mebendazole in patients treated for cystic hydatid disease. Eur J Clin Pharmacol. 1982;22:101–9.

El-Mufti M. Surgical management of hydatid disease. London: Butterworths; 1989.

El-Mufti M, karnag HA, Ibrahim S, Taktuk I, Swaisi AZ. Albendazole therapy of hydatid disease: 2-year follow-up of 40 cases. Ann Trop Med Parasitol. 1993;87(3):241–6.

Evangelos C, et al. Perioperative benzimidazole therapy in human hydatid liver disease. Int Surg. 1995;80:131–3.

French CM. Mebendazole and surgery for human hydatid disease in Turkana. East Afr Med J. 1984;61:113–9.

Heath DD, Christie MJ, Chevisn RAF. The lethal effect of albendazole on secondary Echinococcus granulosus, cysticerici od taeniasis pisiformis and tetrathyridia of mesocestoides corti. Parasitology. 1975;70:273–385.

Horton RJ. Chemotherapyof echinoccoccus infection in man with albendazole. Trans R Soc Trop Med Hyg. 1989;83:97–102.

Khuroo MS. Hydatid disease: current status and recent advances. Ann Saudi Med. 2002;22:56–64.

Little JM, Hollands MT, Eckberg H. Recurrence of hydatid disease. World J Surg. 1988;12:700–70.

Milicevic MN. Hydatid disease. In: Blumgart LH, Fong Y, editors. Surgery of liver and biliary tract. 3rd ed. London: W.B. Saunders; 2000.

Morris DL. Preoperative albendazole therapy for hydatid cyst. Br J Surg. 1987;74:805–6.

Morris DL. Albendazole treatment of hydatid disease: follow up at five years. Trop Doct. 1989;19:179–80.

Morris DL, Gould SE. Serum and cyst concentrations of mebendazole and flubendazole in hydatid disease. Br Med J (Clin Res Ed). 1982;285:175.

Morris DL, Taylor DH. Optimal timing of postoperative albendazole prophylaxis in E. granulosus. Ann Trop Med Parasitol. 1988;82:65–6.

Morris DL, Skeene-Smith H, Haynes A, Burrows FGO. Abdominal hydatid disease: computed tomographic and ultrasound changes during albendazole therapy. Clin Radiol. 1984;35:297–300.

Morris DL, Dykes PW, Marriner S, Bogan J, Burrows F, Skeene-Smith H, Clarkson MJ. Albendazole: objective evidence of response in human hydatid disease. J Am Med Assoc. 1985;253:2053–7.

Morris DL, Chinnery JB, et al. Penetration of albendazole sulphoxide into hydatid cyst. Gut. 1987;28:75–80.

Mottaghion H, Saidi F. Postoperative recurrence of hydayod disease. Br J Surg. 1978;65:237–42.

Okelo GBA. Hydatid disease: research and control in Turkana: III—Albendazole in the treatment of inoperable hydatid disease in Kenya; a report on 12 cases. Trans R Soc Trop Med Hyg. 1986;80:193–5.

Osborne DR. Mebendazole and hydatid disease. Br Med J. 1980;280:183.

Saimot AG, Meulemans A, Cremieux AC, Giovangeli MD, Hay JM, Delaitre B, Coulaund JP. Albendazole as a potential treatment for human hydatidosis. Lancet. 1983;ii:652–6.

Schantz PM, Van den Bossche H, Eckert J. Chemotherapy for larval Echinococcosis in animals and humans. Report of workshop. Zeitschrift fuer Parasitenkunde. 1982;67:5–26.

Sherlock S. Hydatid disease: disease of liver and biliary system. Oxford: Blackwell Scientific; 1981. p. 247–452.

Taylor DH, Morris DL, Richards KS. Combination chemotherapy of *Echinococcus granulosus*—in vitro studies. Trans R Soc Trop Med Hyg. 1988;82:263–4.

Taylor DH, Morris DL, Reffin D, Richards KS. Comparison of albendazole, mebendazole and praziquantel chemotherapy of *Echinococcus multilocularis* in gerbil model. Gut. 1989;30:1401–5.

Wilson JF, Rausch RL. Alveolar hydatid disease; A review of the clinical features of 33 indigenous cases of *Echinococcus multilocularis* Infections in Alaskan Eskimos. Am J Trop Med Hyg. 1980;24:1340–55.

Alveolar Hydatid Disease

Infection caused by larval stage of *E. multilocularis* in humans is less common as compared to *E. granulosus* and is known as alveolar hydatid disease. It is very rare in our part of the world and is mostly seen in Eastern France, Switzerland, Austria, Bulgaria, Turkey, Iran Japan, Afghanistan and Russia (Rausch et al. 1991). It is one of the most life-threatening helminthic infections found in human population. Human beings are unusual and poor intermediate hosts for the *E. multilocularis*, and the disease is usually progressive and destructive in nature (Amir-Jahad et al. 1975; Ammann and Eckert 1996). The growth and proliferation of this larva resembles a slow-growing tumour of the liver and can severely destroy the liver parenchyma and its function. In many situations it may be difficult to differentiate alveolar disease from liver cancer because of infiltration into biliary and vascular tissue of the liver. Early diagnosis and radical surgery is a key to definitive treatment and cure of this fatal disease.

Pathology

The alveolar cysts resulting from the infection with *E. multilocularis* are atypical from that of *E. granulosus*. The high fluid pressure which is found in typical hydatid cysts is absent in the cysts of alveolar hydatid disease (Kantarci et al. 2014). The cyst or metacestode of *E. multilocularis* is thin walled and smaller in size and lacks a definitive capsule. These cysts appear as spongy or gelly-like mass often at the hilum of liver. The cysts are poorly delineated and invade liver tissue just like a malignant disease (Wilson and Rausch 1980). The cyst has many vesicles embedded in a stroma of connective tissue. The growth of parasite is caused by undifferentiated cells of the germinal layer. The lesion is always primary in the liver and proliferates by exogenous growth to form an invasive and infiltrative cancer like growth. Since the favourable tissue is not available in human tissues, the cyst remains in proliferative stage, and protoscoleces are rarely produced. There is usually a surrounding infiltrate of polymorphs, eosinophil's, macrophages and foreign body

© Springer Nature Singapore Pte Ltd. 2019
A. A. Malik, S. Bari, *Human Abdominal Hydatidosis*,
https://doi.org/10.1007/978-981-13-2152-8_6

giant cells. In chronic infections, the lesion consists of a necrotic area in the centre with a thin peripheral rim of dense fibrous tissue, extensively infiltrated by proliferating vesicles (Milicevic 2005).

Life Cycle of *Echinococcus multilocularis*

The life cycle is same as that of *E. granulosus* except that adult worm lives in jejunum of the definitive host (Rohela 2017). *E. multilocularis* is a small cestode, 1.2–4.5 mm in size. Definitive hosts include domestic dogs and cats, wild rodents and wild carnivores such as red fox. The adult worm is characterized by fine proglottids, which reside in jejunum of definitive host. The eggs are released from proglottids of gravid proglottids and are than passed in the faeces to the exterior. Humans and other intermediate hosts get infected by ingestion of food or water contaminated by embryonated eggs (Kantarci et al. 2014) or by directly handling definitive hosts such as cats or dogs or while skinning foxes (Morris and Richards 1992). The major risk of infection in humans occurs when a hunter-pray relationship is established between domestic dogs or cats and wild rodents. The domestic dogs and cats become infected by eating rodents. In such a case, the eggs in faeces of dogs and cats are the major source of infection for humans. In the humans the metacestode, which is a larval stage of parasite develops in liver and is made up of several vesicles which range in size from <1 mm up to 15–20 cm in size (Kantarci et al. 2014). The structure of each vesicle is similar to *E. granulosus* cyst (Stathatos et al. 1986). Sometimes this metacestode can grow rapidly and can cause a serious fatal disease—alveolar echinococcosis. There are no protoscoleces inside the germinative layer of alveolar echinococcosis. However, when these sterile membranes are injected into a live rodents, protoscoleces are produced. *E. multilocularis* is restricted to certain areas of Eastern Europe, Russia, Greece, Iran India and some Japanese Islands.

Immunological Response to *Echinococcus multilocularis*

The parasite induces a strong cellular immune response (Kantarci et al. 2014). Cellular immunity-TH1 cytokine plays a crucial role in defence against the parasite (Ito et al. 1995; Helbig et al. 1993). IL-12 plays a vital role in the induction of TH1 profile. In the liver, the parasitic lesions are formed which are surrounded by a granulomatous infiltrate. The cells involved in the formation of this periparasitic granuloma include macrophages, T-lymphocytes and myofibroblasts (Kantarci et al. 2014). In patients with aggressive disease, high level of TH2 is found, while in patients with progressive disease, increased concentration of IL-4/IL-5 is found. In patients where the parasite has died, a large number of CD4(+) T lymphocytes are found, whereas in patients where the metacestodes are active, there is a significant increase in CD8(+) T cells (Kantarci et al. 2014). This suggests that CD4(+) T cells play a vital role in the killing mechanism. Several mechanisms have been proposed to explain avoidance of *E. granulosus* from host immune responses which include molecular mimicry (Ito et al. 2003), immunomodulation (Ito et al. 2002) and antigen and DNA polymorphism (Harman et al. 2003; Bartholomot et al. 2002).

Clinical Presentation

The liver is the most common site for infection with *E. multilocularis* (Kantarci et al. 2012). The disease has got a non-specific clinical presentation and a very long latency period of 5–15 years. Patients may present with anorexia, mild right upper quadrant abdominal pain (Rohela 2017), weight loss and a palpable abdominal mass or hepatomegaly (Wilson and Rausch 1980). In advanced stage of disease, there will be hepatic insufficiency, ascites and jaundice. The disease may infiltrate into the hepatic veins, and patient can develop a Budd-Chiari syndrome. If the infection is not treated, there is a progressive destruction of liver parenchyma over a period of several years and eventually a death is caused by hepatic failure and invasion into adjacent vital structures with a mortality rate of more than 80%. Various life-threatening complications such as cholangitis, portal hypertension and biliary cirrhosis can develop in patients where the disease invades structures such as bile ducts and blood vessels (Kantarci et al. 2012; Koroglu et al. 2006). After several years of long latent and asymptomatic period, disease can progress to the cirrhotic stage (Sekiya 1994). Involvement of various vital organs such as the liver, brain, lungs and mediastinum can lead to life-threatening complications. Involvement of lungs results in to breathlessness, cough with blood stained sputum and chest pain (Polat et al. 2004). Increased intracranial pressure and epilepsy is seen in patients with brain involvement. Certain neurologic symptoms such as slurred speech, hemiparesis and paralysis of various cranial nerve may also develop in some patients where brain has been involved (Kantarci et al. 2014; Algros et al. 2003). Other complications like abdominal wall involvement and myositis have also been reported. In rare cases, subcutaneous soft tissues and bones may also be involved. The bones which are usually involved are the sternum and vertebrae (Czermak et al. 2001). Involvement of the vertebral column can lead to paresis due to a compression by cysts of alveolar echinococcosis on the spinal cord. Involvement of hollow viscera, ribs and limbs is exceedingly rare (Kantarci et al. 2014).

The international benchmark for standardized evaluation of diagnostic and therapeutic measures based on findings on imaging has been established by the World Health Organization Informal Working Group on Echinococcosis classification system (Kantarci et al. 2012; Sekiya 1994), and the classification has been devised known as PNM system. P indicates the extent of the primary lesion in the liver, N indicates the involvement of adjacent organs including lymph nodes, and M indicates metastases to distant organs (Algros et al. 2003).

PNM System for Classification of Human Alveolar Echinococcosis

P: Hepatic Localisation of the Parasite
PX: Primary lesion cannot be assessed.
P0: No detectable lesion in the liver.
P1: Peripheral lesions without proximal vascular and/or biliary involvement.
P2: Central lesions with proximal vascular and/or biliary involvement of one lobe (a).
P3: Central lesions with hilar vascular and biliary involvement of both lobes and/ or with Involvement of two hepatic veins.
P4: Any liver lesion with extension along the vessels and the biliary tree.

N: Extrahepatic involvement of neighbouring organs (diaphragm, lung, pleura, pericardium, heart, gastric and duodenal wall, adrenal glands, peritoneum, retroperitoneum, parietal wall (muscles, skin, bone), pancreas, regional lymph nodes, liver ligaments, kidney)
NX: Involvement of lymph nodes cannot be evaluated
N0: No regional involvement (see above)
N1: Regional involvement of contiguous organs or tissues

M: Absence or presence of distant metastases (in lung, distant lymph nodes, spleen, CNS, orbital, bone, skin, muscle, distant peritoneum and retroperitoneum).
MX: Presence of distant metastasis cannot be completely evaluated
M0: No metastasis
M1: Metastasis present
(a) For classification, the plane projecting between the bed of the gallbladder and the inferior vena cava divides the liver into two lobes
(b) Vessels refers to inferior vena cava, portal vein and arteries
(c) Chest X-ray and cerebral CT negative.

Diagnosis

The clinical diagnosis of hepatic *E. multilocularis* is based on the history of the patient, clinical features, serological assessment, morphology of lesions at radiological imaging and histopathological features (Kantarci et al. 2012; Koroglu et al. 2006). Diagnosis is based on basis of the presence of at least two of the following three features (Eckert et al. 2000; Koroglu et al. 2006), which include (1) if one or more lesions are present with the typical appearance of alveolar echinococcosis at usual sites on cross-sectional imaging, (2) if serum antibodies specific to *Echinococcus* species are demonstrated in blood tests with further confirmation on immunoassays and (3) if histopathology of specimen suggests features of *E. multilocularis*.

Although in early stages of disease, liver functions are within normal limits, but in advanced stages, the serum bilirubin levels are elevated. Various serological tests have a diagnostic value particularly indirect haemagglutination and ELISA (Wilson and Rausch 1980). However serological tests fail in 5–10% and in such cases results of new PCR techniques are very satisfactory. Certain tests, which are based on the use of Em2, have been found to have a promising role. These include Em2, a species-specific native antigen isolated from the metacestode of *E multilocularis*, and the Em2^{plus} ELISA, which is a combination of Em2 and recombinant protein designated as II/3–10. The serological test, Em2^{plus} ELISA has been widely used for clinical diagnosis and population screening (McManus et al. 2003; Bresson-Hadni et al. 2000; Gottstein et al. 1993; Ito et al. 2002). Em18 (18 kDa antigen) helps to differentiate between live and dead alveolar echinococci. For long-term follow-up of patients put on drug therapy, ELISA with Em2^{plus} and immunostaining with Em18 have been widely used (Ma et al. 1997).

Role of serology is more important in *E. multilocularis* than that of *Echinococcus granulosus*. Immunoelectrophoresis, indirect haemagglutination (IHA) and Arc 5 double diffusion (DD5) have been commonly used, using *E. granulosus* antigens with good results (Schantz et al. 1982). However some patients with *E. multilocularis* will not cross react with *E. granulosus* antigens. Immunological differentiation of *E. granulosus* and *multilocularis* can be done using ELISA (Gottstein et al. 1986). ELISA test in which antigen EM$_2$ is used can help us to know which patients are at risk for getting recurrence after surgery, and such patients can benefit by taking albendazole or mebendazole therapy.

X-ray abdomen shows a diffuse radiolucent areas surrounded by calcification. Ultrasonography, CT abdomen and MRI are useful diagnostic tools and show various morphological changes in the liver and are useful tools to see the extent of disease (Kantarci et al. 2014). Angiography and nuclear scan will show a filling defect (Milicevic 2005). Diagnostic laparoscopy has also been used for evaluation of the disease.

Ultrasonography

Ultrasound of the abdomen is the initial investigation of choice for detection of any hepatic lesions including that of *E. multilocularis* (Koroglu et al. 2006). The typical features are seen in about 70% of patients on ultrasonography. The usual USG features include large hepatic mass in the liver with multiple hyper- and hypo-echoic areas inside the mass. The mass has an indistinct margin with scattered foci of calcification (Kantarci et al. 2012). The other typical feature of alveolar echinococcosis is a pseudocyst formation with a large area of necrosis in the centre surrounded by an irregular ring. This irregular ring is hyper-echoic and represents a fibrous tissue (Kern et al. 2003). In the rest of 30% of cases, multiple clustered haemangioma-like hyper-echoic nodules are seen. These lesions usually have a "hailstorm pattern"

(Kantarci et al. 2014). Histologically, in hailstorm pattern there is heterogeneous stroma containing microscopic metacestode vesicles, areas of non-liquefactive necrosis, entrapped host tissue, and micro-calcifications. The presence of ill-defined borders and calcification and a lack of enhancement of the lesions helps us to differentiate *E. multilocularis* from other liver lesions which usually show enhancement and lack calcification.

On Doppler study, hepatic veins, portal vein and biliary tree are displaced or distorted either due to pressure effect of lesion or invasion of these vital structures by hepatic lesions (Kantarci et al. 2014).

Computed Tomography

Computed tomography is an ideal investigation as it demonstrates the peculiar anatomy and morphology of lesions and typical pattern of calcification (Karçaaltincaba and Sirlin 2011). It provides relevant information regarding the number, size and site of lesions in the liver. It has an important role in preoperative assessment of patients and helps to assess the resectability of lesion with respect to vascular and biliary invasion and extrahepatic extension (Kantarci et al. 2014). On unenhanced CT images, alveolar echinococcosis is seen as an infiltrating lesion with irregular margins and heterogeneous appearance (Figs. 1 and 2). This heterogeneous appearance of the mass is due to scattered hyper-attenuating areas of calcifications and hypo-attenuating areas of necrosis and parasitic tissue (Kantarci et al. 2012). In pseudo cystic type of hepatic lesions, On CT, a large central area of necrosis is seen which is surrounded by an irregular ring of calcification corresponding to fibrous tissue. In patients with hilar infiltration the intrahepatic bile ducts are typically dilated (Kantarci et al. 2014).

Primary hepatic neoplasms such as cholangiocarcinoma, biliary cyst adenoma, biliary cyst adenocarcinoma and hepatic metastases have similar appearance on CT as that of alveolar echinococcosis (Didier et al. 1985; Kantarci et al. 2014). Presence of certain typical radiographic features such as hypo-attenuation, calcification and

Fig. 1 CT image of alveolar echinococcosis of the liver with central necrosis

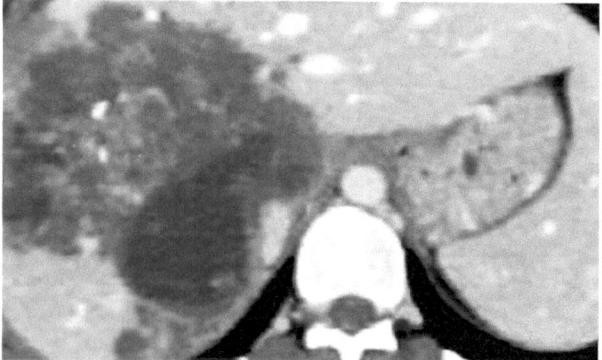

Fig. 2 CT image showing multiple lesions affecting central liver

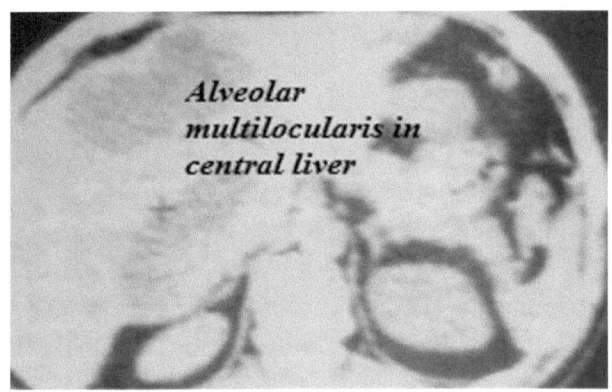

non-enhancement helps us to differentiate them from Echinococcus multilocularis (Karçaaltincaba and Sirlin 2011).

MR Imaging

MRI is the best modality in patients with diagnostic uncertainty as it may show the characteristic multivesicular structure of alveolar echinococcosis lesions and also gives information about the vascular or biliary tree involvement and extrahepatic extension. MRI has a vital role in evaluations of patients who are planned for extensive hepatic resection or liver transplantation as it is very useful in showing extension to adjacent structures (Kantarci et al. 2012; Bresson-Hadni et al. 2006). It is not as helpful as CT in depicting calcification, which is a pathognomonic feature of alveolar echinococcosis.

Features suggestive of alveolar echinococcosis on MRI include an infiltrative mass with heterogeneous appearance with necrosis in the centre and irregular margins that exhibits low to intermediate signal intensity on T1-weighted images and heterogeneous signal intensity on T2-weighted images (Bresson-Hadni et al. 2006). Areas of high T2 signal intensity correspond to small cystic or necrotic components, while as areas with low T2 signal intensity correspond to fibrotic or collagenous components (Kantarci et al. 2012). T2-weighted images are useful for detecting small hepatic cysts and extrahepatic cysts (Kodama et al. 2003; Balci et al. 2000).

Lesions of *E. multilocularis* of liver on MRI are categorized in to five types on the basis of their imaging appearances (Kodama et al. 2003; Kantarci et al. 2012).

- *Type 1*—lesion is composed of multiple small cysts with no solid component.
- *Type 2*—lesion is composed of multiple small cysts with a solid tissue.
- *Type 3*—lesions consist of irregular large cysts along with a solid tissue.
- *Type 4*—lesion is composed of solid tissue with no cystic components.
- *Type 5*—lesion is composed of a single large cyst without any solid components.

Management of Alveolar Echinococcosis

Guidelines for the management of human alveolar disease are in vogue since 1996 and have been updated in 2011 by the WHO Informal Working Group on Echinococcosis (Kantarci et al. 2014). Although the only curative treatment for *E. multilocularis* is the resection of the liver, curative treatment of *E. multilocularis* is possible only in those cases where the disease was detected in early stages and complete surgical excision was possible. As recommended by WHO informal group on echinococcosis 1996 (Guidelines for treatment 1996), all those patients who have been subjected to radical surgery should receive a drug therapy for at least 2 years after complete resection of the lesions (WHO/OIE 2001; Kantarci et al. 2012). If radical surgery was not possible, patient should receive a drug therapy for rest of his life. In all those cases where total resection is possible, radical surgery is the surgery of choice (Kern et al. 2003). Radical resection may be associated with few late complications such as liver abscess, biliary obstruction and portal hypertension. Liver transplantation may be advocated for unresectable patients such as those where the disease is invading deep into the hilum or those with recurrent alveolar echinococcosis (Kantarci et al. 2012). Liver transplantation is also advocated in patients with severe liver dysfunction, symptomatic secondary biliary cirrhosis with ascites and severe oesophageal variceal bleed due to portal hypertension (Harman et al. 2003).

Approximately 93% patients with unresectable disease die within 10 years (Schantz et al. 1982). If surgery is not possible, various interventional procedures can be attempted which include percutaneous bile drainage or drainage of pus and endoscopic dilation of bile duct strictures followed by insertion of plastic stents. Some authors advocate a palliative surgery with or without chemotherapy (Kantarci et al. 2012; Bhatia et al. 2016).

There is no current consensus as far as the treatment of cerebral lesions is concerned (Kantarci et al. 2014). However whenever possible, surgery is always preferred, and when a surgical approach is not possible, procedures such as cerebrospinal fluid shunt surgery, γ knife radiosurgery or drug therapy with anthelminthic and anti-inflammatory drugs are the options available (Polat et al. 2004).

Drug Therapy in *Echinococcus multilocularis*

Benzimidazole group of antibiotics have been widely used with varied results. Early reports with mebendazole were promising as was shown by Bekhti et al. (1977). These drugs block the transport of secretory substances and uptake of glucose and cause degeneration of the germinative layer, inadequate nutrition and autolysis. It has been reported that although mebendazole does not kill the parasite, it does stop further progression of disease (Wilson and Rausch 1980).

Mebendazole in dose of 40–50 mg/kg has been found to give symptomatic relief in patients with unresectable disease and also improve survival and decrease recurrence in patients with resectable disease (Wilson and Rausch 1980). The principal metabolite of albendazole (sulphoxide) has been found to be active against protoscoleces of *E. multilocularis* in various studies (Taylor and Morris 1988). The effectiveness of combination of albendazole and praziquantel was initially studied in animals and in vitro cultures (Taylor and Morris 1989). Albendazole in dose of 50 mg/kg has been found to be more effective than mebendazole 50 mg/kg and praziquantel 500 mg kg per day (Horton 1989). However some have questioned the efficacy of albendazole (Schantz et al. 1982). Combinations of different benzimidazole have yet not been evaluated. Use of ivermectin in combination with praziquantel in alveolar *Echinococcus* is being studied. The effect of hyperthermia in combination with chemotherapy on *E. multilocularis* has been found to be useful in experimental studies (Ito et al. 1995).

References

Algros MP, Majo F, Bresson-Hadni S, et al. Intracerebral alveolar echinococcosis. Infection. 2003;31(1):63–5.

Amir-Jehad AK, Faria R, Furzad R. Clinical echinococcus. Ann Surg. 1975;182:541–5.

Ammann RW, Eckert J. Cestodes: echinococcus. Gastroenterol Clin North Am. 1996;25(3):655–89.

Balci NC, Tunaci A, Semelka RC, et al. Hepatic alveolar echinococcosis: MRI findings. Magn Reson Imaging. 2000;18(5):537–41.

Bartholomot G, Vuitton DA, Harraga S, et al. Combined ultrasound and serologic screening for hepatic alveolar echinococcosis in central China. Am J Trop Med Hyg. 2002;66(1):23–9.

Bekhti A, Schaaps JP, Capron M, Dessaint JP, Santoro F, Capron A. Treatment of hepatic hydatid disease with mebendazole: preliminary results in four cases. Br Med J. 1977;ii:1047–51.

Bhatia JK, Ravikumar R, Naidu CS, Sethumadhavan T. Alveolar hydatid disease of the liver: a rare entity in India. Med J Armed Forces India. 2016;72(1):S126–9.

Bresson-Hadni S, Vuitton DA, Bartholomot B, et al. A twenty-year history of alveolar echinococcosis: analysis of a series of 117 patients from eastern France. Eur J Gastroenterol Hepatol. 2000;12(3):327–36.

Bresson-Hadni S, Delabrousse E, Blagosklonov O, et al. Imaging aspects and non-surgical interventional treatment in human alveolar echinococcosis. Parasitol Int. 2006;55(Suppl):S267–72.

Czermak BV, Unsinn KM, Gotwald T, et al. *Echinococcus multilocularis* revisited. AJR Am J Roentgenol. 2001;176(5):1207–12.

Didier D, Weiler S, Rohmer P, et al. Hepatic alveolar echinococcosis: correlative US and CT study. Radiology. 1985;154(1):179–86.

Eckert J, Conraths FJ, Tackmann K. Echinococcosis: an emerging or re-emerging zoonosis? Int J Parasitol. 2000;30(12–13):1283–94.

Gottstein B, Schantz PM, Todoro VT, et al. An international study on the serological differentiation of human cyst and alveolar Echinococcus after complete surgical resection of liver lesion. Trans R Soc Trop Med Hyg. 1986;83:389–93.

Gottstein B, Jacquier P, Bresson-Hadni S, Eckert J. Improved primary immunodiagnosis of alveolar echinococcosis in humans by an enzyme-linked immunosorbent assay using the Em2plus antigen. J Clin Microbiol. 1993;31(2):373–6.

Guidelines for treatment of cystic and alveolar echinococcosis in humans. WHO Informal Working Group on echinococcosis. Bull World Health Organ. 1996;74(3):231–42.

Harman M, Arslan H, Kotan C, Etlik O, Kayan M, Deveci A. MRI findings of hepatic alveolar echinococcosis. Clin Imaging. 2003;27(6):411–6.

Helbig M, Frosch P, Kern P, Frosch M. Serological differentiation between cystic and alveolar echinococcosis by use of recombinant larval antigens. J Clin Microbiol. 1993;31(12):3211–5.

Horton RJ. Chemotherapy of *Echinococcus* infection in man with albendazole. Trans R Soc Trop Med Hyg. 1989;87:97–102.

Ito A, Schantz PM, Wilson JF. Em18, a new serodiagnostic marker for differentiation of active and inactive cases of alveolar hydatid disease. Am J Trop Med Hyg. 1995;52(1):41–4.

Ito A, Xiao N, Liance M, et al. Evaluation of an enzyme-linked immunosorbent assay (ELISA) with affinity-purified Em18 and an ELISA with recombinant Em18 for differential diagnosis of alveolar echinococcosis: results of a blind test. J Clin Microbiol. 2002;40(11):4161–5.

Ito A, Sako Y, Yamasaki H, et al. Development of Em18-immunoblot and Em18-ELISA for specific diagnosis of alveolar echinococcosis. Acta Trop. 2003;85(2):173–82.

Kantarci M, Bayraktutan U, Karabulut N, Aydinili B, Ogul H, Yuce I, Calik M, Eren S, Atamanlap SS, Ota A. Alveolar echinococcosis: spectrum of findings at cross sectional imaging. Radiographics. 2012;32(7):2053–70.

Kantarci M, Pirimoglu B, Kizrak Y. Diagnostic imaging and interventional procedures in a growing problem: hepatic alveolar echinococcosis. World J Surg Proced. 2014;4(1):13–20.

Karçaaltincaba M, Sirlin CB. CT and MRI of diffuse lobar involvement pattern in liver pathology. Diagn Interv Radiol. 2011;17(4):334–42.

Kern P, Bardonnet K, Renner E, et al. European echinococcosis registry: human alveolar echinococcosis, Europe, 1982–2000. Emerg Infect Dis. 2003;9(3):343–9.

Kodama Y, Fujita N, Shimizu T, et al. Alveolar echinococcosis: MR findings in the liver. Radiology. 2003;228(1):172–7.

Koroglu M, Akhan O, Gelen MT, et al. Complete resolution of an alveolar echinococcosis liver lesion following percutaneous treatment. Cardiovasc Intervent Radiol. 2006;29(3):473–8.

Ma L, Ito A, Liu YH, et al. *Alveolar echinococcosis*: Em2plus-ELISA and Em18-western blots for follow-up after treatment with albendazole. Trans R Soc Trop Med Hyg. 1997;91(4):476–8.

McManus DP, Zhang W, Li J, Bartley PB. Echinococcosis. Lancet. 2003;362(9392):1295–304.

Milicevic MN. Hydatid disease. In: Blumgart LH, Fong Y, editors. Surgery of liver and biliary tract. 3rd ed. London: W.B. Saunders; 2005.

Morris DL, Richards KS. Hydatid disease; current medical and surgical management. Jordon Hill Oxford: Butterworth –Heinemann Ltd; 1992. p. 1167–97.

Polat KY, Ozturk G, Aydinli B, Kantarci M. Images of interest: hepatobiliary and pancreatic: alveolar hydatid disease. J Gastroenterol Hepatol. 2004;19(11):1319.

Rausch RL, Wilson JF, Schwartz PM. A program to reduce risk of infection by *Echinococcus multilocularis*: use of praziquantel to control the cestode in a village in the hyperendemic region of Alaska. Ann Trop Med Parasitol. 1991;84:239–50.

Rohela Mahmud, Yvonne Ai Lian Lim, Amirah Amir. Cestodes; Tapeworms. Medical Parasitology. 2017, p. 117–34.

Schantz PM, Van den Bossche H, Eckert J. Chemotherapy for larval echinococcosis in animals and humans. Report of workshop. Zeitschrift Fuer Parasitenkunde. 1982;67:5–26.

Sekiya C. Parasitic cirrhosis of the liver [in Japanese]. Nihon Rinsho. 1994;52(1):234–9.

Stathatos C, Kontaxis A, Zaphiracopoulos P. Hydatid cyst of the liver. Sixth Panhellenic Congress of Surgery VI. 1986: 365.

Taylor DH, Moris DL. In vitro culture of Echinococcus multilocularis :protoscolicidal action of praziquantal and albendazole sulphoxide. Trans R Soc Trop Med Hyg. 1988;82:265–7.

Taylor DH, Morris DL. Combination chemotherapy is more effective in post spillage prophylaxis for hydatid disease than either albendazole or praziquantal alone. Br J Surg. 1989;76:954.

WHO/OIE manual on echinococcosis in humans and animals: a public health problem of global concern. Paris: WHO/OIE; 2001.

Wilson JF, Rausch RL. Alveolar hydatid disease; A review of the clinical features of 33 indigenous cases of *Echinococcus multilocularis* infections in Alaskan eskimos. Am J Trop Med Hyg. 1980;24:1340–55.

Primary Splenic Hydatidosis

Primary splenic hydatidosis is defined as the presence of isolated splenic hydatid cysts in absence of such cysts in any other part of the body. It is an uncommon condition accounting for about 2% of the overall hydatid disease burden. Spleen is the third most common organ to be affected by the disease after liver and the lungs (Amr et al. 1994; Shukla et al. 1991).

Etiology

Hydatid disease is caused by parasite *Echinococcus*. *Echinococcus* belongs to the phylum Platyhelminthes (tapeworms). Human echinococcosis is caused by four known species of *Echinococcus*, namely, *Echinococcus granulosus*, *E. multilocularis*, *E. vogeli* and *E. oligarthus*. Only the former three are of medical importance. *E. granulosus* causes cystic echinococcosis, whereas *E. multilocularis* causes alveolar echinococcosis. *E. multilocularis* is rare and the most virulent, while as *E. vogeli* is the most rare species among all. The life cycle of *Echinococcus* involves two hosts, a definitive host and an intermediate host. Definitive hosts include wolf foxes, hyenas, jackals and dogs, while the intermediate hosts include camels, pigs, sheep, cattle, goats, horses and many other animals. Humans act as an accidental intermediate host.

The life cycle has three developmental stages:

– The adult tapeworm in the definitive host
– Eggs in the environment
– The metacestode in the intermediate host

Metacestodes are taken by the definitive host. The metacestodes then mature into the tapeworm in the definitive host. The adult tapeworms release eggs into the environment which are taken by the intermediate host. These eggs hatch into metacestodes in the gut of the intermediate host and then infest the liver, lungs, muscles and

© Springer Nature Singapore Pte Ltd. 2019
A. A. Malik, S. Bari, *Human Abdominal Hydatidosis*,
https://doi.org/10.1007/978-981-13-2152-8_7

other organs. Exposure to food and water contaminated by the feces of an infected definitive host can lead to echinococcosis.

Pathophysiology

Once the contaminated food is taken by humans, hexacanth embryos reach the liver via portal circulation. As a result, majority of the hydatid cysts develop in the liver. However some hexacanths escape the hepatic filter and reach to the lungs after passing through the heart. Splenic hydatidosis occurs in those cases where the hexacanths return to the heart from lungs and then enter the systemic circulation leading to dissemination to other extrahepatic extrapulmonary organs. Splenic involvement may occur directly following lymphatic spread from the gut into the systemic circulation (Singh and Arora 2003), or due to reflux from portal vein (Kireşi et al. 2003), at the time of raised intraabdominal pressure. Primary and exclusive involvement of spleen is rare. Primary involvement of the spleen usually occurs due to spread of disease through the arterial blood after the parasite has bypassed the liver and lungs (Malik et al. 2011).

Epidemiology

Echinococcosis remains an endemic disease in Mediterranean countries, the Middle East, Central Asia China, the southern part of South America, Iceland, Australia, New Zealand and southern parts of Africa (Amr et al. 1994). No sexual predilection is recognized for hydatid cysts. The cysts grow slowly. Cystic echinococcosis is a disease of younger adults, average age at diagnosis of 30–40 years, whereas alveolar echinococcosis affects older adults, with an average age at diagnosis of older than 50 years (Uriarte et al. 1991).

Clinical Presentation

The splenic hydatidosis can be seen in both males and females in equal proportion. Most of the splenic cysts are asymptomatic and are incidentally discovered as splenomegaly (Santosh et al. 2017; Varghese and Balakrishnan 1979). Non-specific symptoms like dull dragging sensation, left upper abdominal lump, dyspepsia, constipation and dyspnea due to pushing up of the left diaphragm are usually present (Mills 1924; Alfageme et al. 1994). Some patients may present with complications such as infection of the cyst, intraperitoneal rupture of the cyst and fistula formation into hollow viscera like the colon or stomach followed by upper or lower gastrointestinal bleeding (Santosh et al. 2017; Bitton et al. 1992). Others may present with sympathetic pleural effusion, calcification (Arikanoglu et al. 2012), hypersplenism (Kune and Morris 1990), broncho-pleural fistula and severe urticaria (Lewall and McCorkell 1986).

Diagnosis

The blood counts are usually normal. Eosinophilia (above 3%) is the most common laboratory finding. Ultrasonography and computed tomography scan are the mainstay imaging techniques for diagnosis and screening (Fig. 1). They are non-specific since similar radiographic features may be seen in other cystic lesions of spleen, such as abscess, hematoma, epidermoid cyst, pseudocyst formation or neoplasms (Durgun et al. 2003). However but in combination with serology in combination with radiography has a sensitivity of more than 90%.

Serological diagnosis is commonly employed. Serum immunoelectrophoresis has a sensitivity of approximately 90%. However its main disadvantage is that titres of antibody remain high even 1 year after the infection has been eliminated. Although the sensitivity of indirect haemagglutination test is 85%, it remains positive for several years (Ammann and Eckert 1996).

Plain X-ray of the abdomen findings are usually non-specific and may show a soft tissue shadow with or without an egg shell calcification in the left upper quadrant (Fig. 2). The left hemi-diaphragm, stomach or transverse colon may be displaced from their respective positions. The downward displacement of splenic flexure is considered as a pathognomonic feature of splenic enlargement (Singh and Arora 2003). Intravenous urography may also give some clue as it may show displacement of kidney inferiorly.

Fig. 1 CT image of hydatid spleen

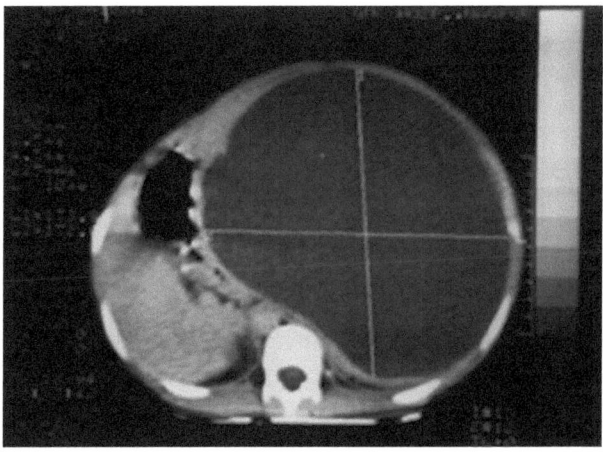

Fig. 2 X-ray abdomen with a calcified soft tissue shadow calcification in the left upper quadrant—hydatid spleen

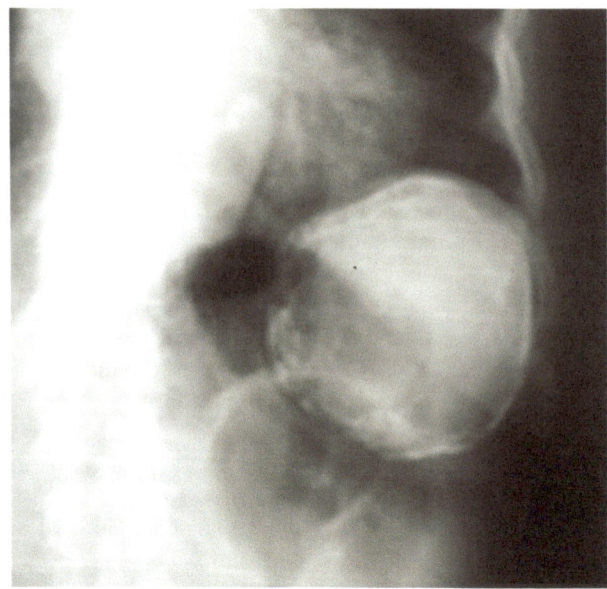

Fig. 3 Postoperative photograph of specimen of spleen with intact hydatid cyst

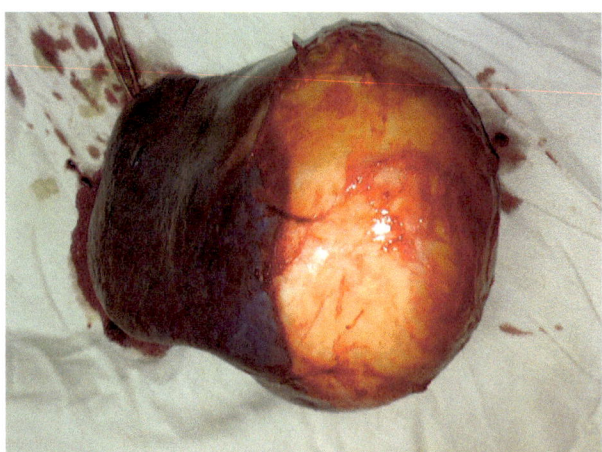

Treatment

The treatment is principally surgical. Splenectomy is the treatment of choice for splenic hydatid cysts (Amman Safioleas et al. 1997; Wani et al. 2005; Malik et al. 2011) as it is an effective mode of treatment for elimination of disease (Fig. 3). Conservative surgical methods such as partial splenectomy, enucleation of the cyst, deroofing of the cyst followed by omentoplasty or external drainage can be done for superficial cysts, cysts located in one pole of the spleen or cysts which are unresectable due to huge size and perisplenic adhesions (Ran et al. 2014). In order to kill the daughter cysts and thereby preventing further spread, recurrence and anaphylactic reaction scolicidal agents such as hypertonic saline or 0.5% silver nitrate is instilled into the cyst before opening the cyst (Malik et al. 2011).

Pre- and postoperative administration of albendazole for a period of 1 month is used to sterilize the cyst, to reduce the risk of anaphylaxis and to reduce the postoperative recurrence rate. Newer techniques like percutaneous aspiration, injection and re-aspiration (Akhan et al. 2016) and laparoscopic evacuation (Khoury et al. 2000) are being increasingly employed and have been found to be safe and effective.

References

Akhan O, Akkaya S, Dağoğlu MG, et al. Percutaneous treatment of splenic cystic echinococcosis: results of 12 cases. Cardiovasc Intervent Radiol. 2016;39:441.

Alfageme I, Martin M, Hernandez J, Huertas C. Rupture of a long-standing splenic hydatid cyst into the bronchial tree. Clin Infect Dis. 1994;19:992–4.

Amman Safioleas M, Misiakos E, Manti C. Surgical treatment for splenic hydatidosis. World J Surg. 1997;21:374–89.

Ammann RW, Eckert J. Cestodes. Echinococcus. Gastroenterol Clin North Am. 1996;25:655–89.

Amr SS, Amr ZS, Jitwani S. Hydatidosis in Jordan: an epidemiological study of 306 cases. Ann Trop Med Parasitol. 1994;88:623–7.

Arikanoglu Z, Taskesen F, Gumus H, Onder A, Aliosmanoglu I, Gul M, et al. Selecting a surgical modality to treat a splenic hydatid cyst: total splenectomy or spleen-saving surgery? J Gastrointest Surg. 2012;16:1189–93.

Bitton M, Kleiner-Baumgarten A, Peiser J, Barki Y, Sukenik S. Anaphylactic shock after traumatic rupture of a splenic echinococcal cyst. Harefuah. 1992;122:226–8.

Durgun V, Kapan S, Kapan M, Karabiçak I, Aydogan F, Goksoy E. Primary splenic hydatidosis. Dig Surg. 2003;20:38–41.

Khoury G, Abiad F, Geagea T, Nabout G, Jabbour S. Laparoscopic treatment of hydatid cysts of the liver and spleen. Surg Endosc. 2000;14:243–5.

Kireşi DA, Karabacakoğlu A, Odev K, Karaköse S. Uncommon locations of hydatid cysts. Acta Radiol. 2003;44:622–36.

Kune GA, Morris DL. Hydatid disease. In: Schwartz SI, Ellis H, editors. Maingots abdominal operations. London: Appleton and Lange; 1990. p. 1225–40.

Lewall DB, McCorkell SJ. Rupture of echinococcal cysts: diagnosis, classification, and clinical implications. AJR Am J Roentgenol. 1986;146:391–4.

Malik AA, Bari SUL, Younis M. Primary splenic hydatidosis. Indian J Gastroenterol. 2011;30(4):175–17.

Mills HW. Hydatid cyst of the spleen, with report of four cases. Gynaec Obst. 1924;38:491–505.

Ran B, Shao Y, Yimiti Y, Aji T, Shayiding P, Jiang T, et al. Spleen Preserving surgery is effective for the treatment of spleen cystic echinococcosis. Int J Infect Dis. 2014;29:181–3.

Santosh T, Patro MK, Bal AK, Behera B. Hydatid cyst at unusual locations. Report of two cases. Hum Pathol Case Rep. 2017;8:59–61.

Shukla RA, Hathia WP, Dadhagara KM. Hydatid disease in Saurashtra study of 210 cases. In: Saksena DS, Jhawar DK, Purohit A, editors. Surgery in the tropics. New Delhi: Macmillan India; 1991. p. 450–60.

Singh H, Arora S. Primary hydatid cyst of spleen. MJAFI. 2003;5:169–70.

Uriarte C, Pomares N, Martin M, Conde A, Alonso N, Bueno MG. Splenic hydatidosis. Am J Trop Med Hyg. 1991;44(4):420–3.

Varghese C, Balakrishnan V. Hydatid cyst of spleen: an unusual presentation. J Assoc Phys India. 1979;27:1039–41.

Wani RA, Malik AA, Chowdri NA, Wani KA. Primary enterohepatic abdominal hydatidosis. Int J Surg. 2005;3:125–7.

Hydatid Disease of the Kidney

Hydatid disease of kidney is extremely rare and constitutes only 2–3% of all cases and usually associated with hydatid disease of liver or lungs (Diamond et al. 1976). Primary hydatid disease of kidney without the involvement of the liver and lungs is even rarer (Gogus et al. 2003). The age of the patients is 30 and 50 years (Aragona et al. 1984). The cyst is usually single and lies in the cortex of the kidney (Poulios 1991). The symptoms depend on the size and extent of the cyst. These cysts may reach an enormous size before becoming symptomatic (Poulios 1991). Patients may be asymptomatic if the cyst is closed but are symptomatic if it is communicating with the pelvis. In majority of patients, a palpable mass is the only clinical sign (Halim and Vaezzadeh 1980; Baxter-Smith et al. 1987). Clinically, renal hydatid cysts may remain asymptomatic for many years or may present with lumbar pain, haematuria, intermittent fever or hypertension (Haines et al. 1977; Handa and Harjai 2005).

The diagnosis of renal hydatid disease is suggested by passage of hydatid membranes or daughter cysts in urine, known as hydatiduria, which is a pathognomonic feature although, macroscopic hydatiduria is rarely documented (Afsar et al. 1991, 1994). Microscopic hydatiduria may be seen in 10–20% of cases of renal hydatidosis (Kiresi et al. 2003). It is characterized by an episode of renal colic followed by passage of grapelike material in the urine. The specific diagnosis of hydatid disease can be made by identifying protoscoleces or hooklets in cyst fluid, although fluid aspiration is not recommended due to risk of fluid leakage and anaphylaxis reaction (Reddy et al. 1968). Saline mount, modified Baxby staining procedure and haematoxylin and eosin staining can be done on cyst fluid for better visualization of hooklets.

Pathogenesis

Although exact route of spread of the hydatid embryo to the kidney in case of primary hydatid disease is not known, it is postulated that it passes through the portal system into the liver and from there it reaches to the kidney through retroperitoneal

© Springer Nature Singapore Pte Ltd. 2019
A. A. Malik, S. Bari, *Human Abdominal Hydatidosis*,
https://doi.org/10.1007/978-981-13-2152-8_8

lymphatics (Gogus et al. 1991). Those hydatid cysts of the kidney where all the three layers, i.e. pericyst, ectocyst and endocyst, are intact are known as a closed cyst. On the other hand, when the third layer is absent or cyst is protected by the lining of collecting system only, it is said to be an exposed cyst. In an open cyst also known as a communicating cyst, all the three layers of the cyst have ruptured with the resultant free communication with the pelvi-calcyeal system. This rupture of the cyst into the collecting system causes hydatiduria. It is a pathognomonic feature of renal hydatidosis seen in only 10–20% of renal hydatidosis and is usually micro-scopic (Von Lictenberg and Lehman 1978). Gross passage is uncommon, but if there is gross passage, it is undoubtedly diagnostic feature of kidney hydatidosis. The cysts passed in the urine are typically daughter cysts and lack the third layer pericyst, which is otherwise contributed by the host around the mother cyst (Cirenei et al. 1997).

Investigations

Results of blood cell counts and blood chemistry are non-specific except for eosino-philia which may be seen in about 50% of cases. Serology and imaging studies have a specific role in the diagnosis of disease (Gharde et al. 2012; Shah et al. 2009). Although various serological tests such as immunoelectrophoresis, immunohemag-glutination test and complement fixation test are very helpful in diagnosis, the enzyme-linked immunosorbent assay (ELISA) and polymerase chain reaction (PCR) are widely used. In primary renal hydatidosis serological tests are usually negative.

Radiologic tests are important tools for the diagnosis of renal hydatid disease. USG and computed tomography (CT) scan are the common imaging modalities for the diagnosis of renal hydatid disease (Shah et al. 2009). CT scan has advantage over USG as it can easily detect calcifications and daughter cysts and is more sensi-tive and accurate (Hakami et al. 1993; Horchani et al. 1983).

Plain X-ray films are usually non-specific and may not help much in diagnosis. Plain X-ray film may show a soft tissue mass in the renal area with or without calci-fication. If calcification is present, it is generally peripheral curvilinear and eggshell like (Hertz et al. 1984). Intravenous urography shows a calcified renal cyst. In case a daughter cyst is communicating with the collecting system, it can be outlined.

Ultrasonography

The accuracy of ultrasound evaluation remains operator-dependent. On USG, hyda-tid cyst of kidney appears as a unilocular or multilocular cyst as is the case with hydatid cyst of liver. The endocyst may get detached inside the cavity which is highly specific for hydatid disease and is known as "water lily sign". Multivesicular cysts appear as well-defined fluid collections in a honeycomb pattern, with multiple septa representing the walls of the daughter cysts separated by the hydatid matrix, consistent with spokes of wheel, known as cartwheel pattern. The detached membrane containing vesicle and scoleces may precipitate to the bottom of the hydatid fluid and is known as hydatid sand. Ultrasonography helps in the diagnosis of hydatid cysts in those cases where daughter cysts and hydatid sand is present within the cystic lesion. When the position of patient is changed during USG examination, there is shifting of hydatid sand giving rise to the "falling snowflake pattern". Ring-like or total calcification can be seen during the natural evolution which is commonly seen in hydatid disease of the liver, spleen and kidney (Mongha et al. 2008; Shukla et al. 2011). If a hydatid cyst ruptures into the collecting system, the disease can spread to the ureters or bladder (Gilsanz et al. 1980; Pinar et al. 2003).

Computed Tomography

The CT scan has an accuracy of 98% and has got high sensitivity in demonstrating the daughter cysts. On CT scan renal hydatid cyst is usually seen as an expansile, hypo-attenuating tumour with a well-defined wall and daughter cysts within it (Figs. 1 and 2). The central cystic part of the lesion has got high attenuating value

Fig. 1 CT image of multiloculated hydatid cyst of right kidney

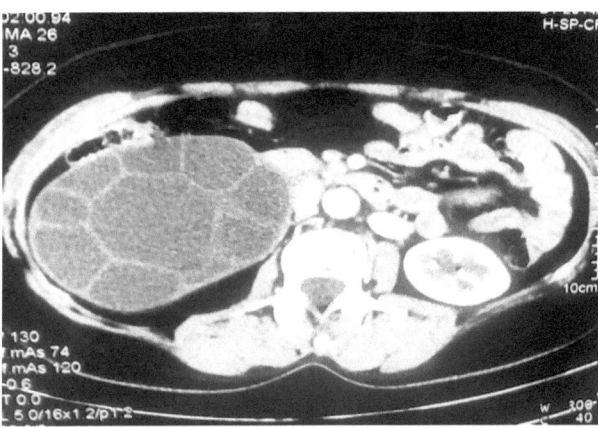

Fig. 2 CT image of hydatid cyst of left kidney

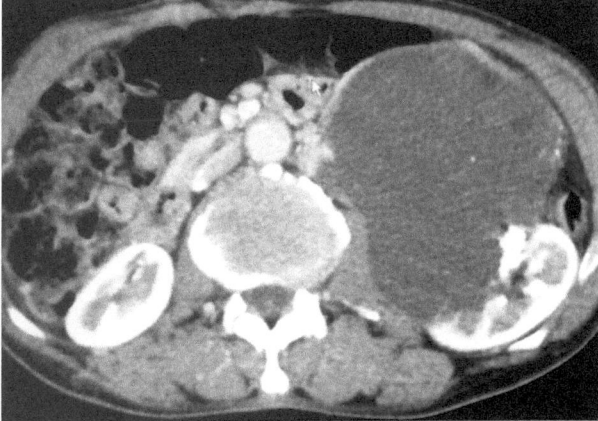

of 30–35 HU, while the fluid in the surrounding cysts has got much lower attenuation value of 5–15 HU, giving the mass a wheel-like or rosette appearance (Amin et al. 2009).

Magnetic Resonance Imaging

Although, the cysts are adequately seen on magnetic resonance imaging (MRI), but it offers no real advantage over CT scan (Pinar et al. 2003). On MRI renal hydatid cyst is seen as a solitary, high-signal-intensity mass consisting of multiple thin-walled lesions outlined by a thick, hypo-intense rim. The high signal intensity is due to the characteristic high fluid content of the mass. The small peripheral cysts are usually hypo-intense relative to the central component (Pinar et al. 2003).

Treatment

Surgery is the treatment of choice in renal hydatid cyst and kidney sparing surgery is possible in 75% of cases (Cirenei et al. 1997; Cushieri et al. 2000). In 75% of the cases, kidney sparing surgery can be done which consists of the cystectomy or pericystectomy with ablation of the hydatid membrane and of small vesicles (Rami et al. 2011; Hakami et al. 1993). Utmost care should be taken during the surgery to prevent spillage and resultant disseminated hydatidosis. Superficial renal hydatid cysts that do not involve the renal parenchyma can be treated by cystectomy or pericystectomy (Tryfonas et al. 1993). However, in those cases where the cyst extends deep into the renal parenchyma, partial nephrectomy can be performed (Beyribey et al. 1995). An attempt must be always made to preserve as much of the parenchyma as possible to maintain the function of the kidney. Nephrectomy may be needed in as many as 25% cases (Shah et al. 2009) and is the treatment of choice for complicated renal hydatid cysts such as those where the cyst is communicating with the ureter, those with seeding in multiple areas and completely destroyed kidney or where the whole kidney is replaced by the cyst where partial removal can lead to relapse and incomplete cure.

Percutaneous management of renal hydatid cyst has been reported in literature and is considered to be a safe option (Goel et al. 1995). PAIR (puncture, aspiration, injection of scolicidal agent, re-aspiration) technique under USG guidance can be an alternative treatment for renal hydatid cysts that are located away from the collecting system of the kidney. It is also useful in cases in which the renal parenchyma needs to be preserved. The disadvantages of this method include dissemination of daughter cysts and fatal anaphylaxis (Buckley et al. 1985).

Laparoscopic removal of renal hydatid has also been reported, and more and more surgeons are attempting with the increasing experience in laparoscopic surgery. However there are high chances of cyst rupture, dissemination, and incomplete removal of the hydatid cyst (Basiri et al. 2006). Both transperitoneal and retroperitoneal laparoscopic management of renal hydatid has been reported (Malik et al. 2007;

Khan et al. 2010; Ozden et al. 2011). The transperitoneal approach is considered superior because it provides a better working space outside the Gerota fascia and prevents subsequent cyst rupture (Shah et al. 2009; Divarci et al. 2010). Laparoscopic transperitoneal nephrectomy can be performed for cases in which the kidney is totally replaced by the hydatid cyst (Shah et al. 2009). In cases in which the cyst is located at one pole of the kidney, laparoscopic partial nephrectomy is the preferred approach because it preserves the normal renal parenchyma (Kumar et al. 2008). Laparoscopic cystopericystectomy is another option that has been described in the literature, and two cases have been reported so far (Beyribey et al. 1995; Bilen et al. 2006). Laparoscopic transperitoneal aspiration of the cyst, followed by deroofing of the cyst wall and endocyst removal, has also been reported (Prabhudessai et al. 2009).

Drug Therapy in Renal Hydatid

Although albendazole therapy has been used widely in the treatment of liver and lung hydatid disease, no data are available on the efficacy of medical treatment in patients with renal hydatid cysts. Albendazole can be used both preoperatively and postoperatively in patients with renal hydatid disease. The aim of using albendazole therapy is to sterilize the cyst; decrease the incidence of anaphylactic reaction; reduce the tension in the cyst wall, thereby preventing spillage and anaphylaxis; and decrease the postoperative recurrence rate (Shukla et al. 2011; Amin et al. 2009). Albendazole therapy is a treatment of choice in patients with disseminated hydatid disease, localized disease with poor surgical risk, ruptured cysts and significant intraoperative spillage.

References

Afsar H, Sanal I, Bayram MM. Renal hydatid disease with hydatiduria. Gaziantep Universitesi Tip Fakultesi Dergisi. 1991;2:201–4.
Afsar H, Yagci F, Aybasti N, Meto S. Hydatid disease of the kidney. Br J Urol. 1994;73:17–21.
Amin MU, Siddique K, Aftab PA. Imaging features of renal hydatid cyst presenting with hydatiduria. J Radiol Case Rep. 2009;3:6–11.
Aragona F, Di Candio G, Serretta V, Fiorentini L. Renal hydatid disease: report of 9 cases and discussion of urological diagnostic procedures. Urol Radiol. 1984;6:182–6.
Basiri A, Nadjafi-Semnani M, Nooralizadeh A. Laparoscopic partial nephrectomy for isolated renal hydatid disease. J Endourol. 2006;20(1):24–8.
Baxter-Smith DC, Smith SET, Hughes MA. Renal hydatid disease: an usual aetiology. Br J Urol. 1987;60:179.
Beyribey S, Cetinkaya M, Adsan O, et al. Treatment of renal hydatid disease by pedicled omentoplasty. J Urol. 1995;154(1):25–7.
Bilen CY, Ozkaya O, Sarıkaya S, Aşci R, Buyukalpelli R. Laparoscopic excision of renal hydatid cyst in a preadolescent. J Pediatr Urol. 2006;2:210–3.
Buckley RJ, Smith S, Herschorn S, Comisarow RH, Barkin M. Echinococcal disease of kidney presenting as renal filling defect. J Urol. 1985;133:660–1.
Cirenei A. Histopathology, clinical findings and treatment of renal hydatidosis. Ann Ital Chir. 1997;68:275–84.

Cushieri A, Steele RJC, Moosa AR. Treatment of hydatid cyst, Essential surgical practice. 4th ed. London: Arnold; 2000.

Diamond HM, Lyon ES, Hui NT, De Pauw AP. Echinococcal disease of kidney. J Urol. 1976;115:742–4.

Divarci E, Ulman I, Avanoglu A. Retroperitoneoscopic laparoscopic treatment of renal hydatid cyst in a child. J Pediatr Surg. 2010;45:262–4.

Gharde P, Wagh DD, Patil A. Left renal hydatid cyst presenting as hematuria and macroscopic hydatiduria since last ten years. Trop Parasitol. 2012;2:58–60.

Gilsanz V, Lozano F, Jimenez J. Renal hydatid cysts: communicating with collecting system. AJR Am J Roentgenol. 1980;135:357–61.

Goel MC, Agarwal MR, Misra A. Percutaneous drainage of renal hydatid cyst: early results and follow-up. Br J Urol. 1995;75:724–8.

Gogus O, Beduk Y, Topukcu Z. Renal hydatid disease. Br J Urol. 1991;68:466–9.

Gogus CM, Safak M, Baltaci S, Turkolmez K. Isolated renal hydatidosis: experience with 20 cases. J Urol. 2003;169(1):186–9.

Haines JG, Mayo ME, Allan TNK, Ansell JS. Echinococcal cyst of kidney. J Urol. 1977;117:788–9.

Hakami F, Tourneur G, Dahern F, Dahmani G, Devoldere H, Abourachid H. Kyste hydatique du rein, Apport de l'imagerie. Progrès en Urologie. 1993;3(1):61–5.

Halim A, Vaezzadeh K. Hydatid disease of genitourinary tract. Br J Urol. 1980;52:75–8.

Handa R, Harjai MM. Hydatid cyst of the renal pelvis. Pediatr Surg Int. 2005;21:410–2.

Hertz M, Zissin R, Dresnik Z, Morag B, Itzchak Y, Jonas P. Echinococcus of the urinary tract: radiologic findings. Urol Radiol. 1984;6:175–81.

Horchani A, Hassine W, Gharbi HA, Saied A, Ayed M, Zmerli S. Apport de l'échographie dans le diagnostic du kyste hydatique de rein: à propos de 43 cas vérifiés. J Urol. 1983;89(7):515–20.

Khan M, Sajjad Nazir S, Ahangar S, Farooq Qadri SJ, Ahmad Salroo N. Retroperitoneal laparoscopy for the management of renal hydatid cyst. Int J Surg. 2010;8:266–8.

Kiresi DA, Karabacakoglu A, Odev K, Karakose S. Uncommon locations of hydatid cysts. Acta Radiol. 2003;44:622–36.

Kumar S, Pandya S, Agarwal S, Lal A. Laparoscopic management of genitourinary hydatid cyst disease. J Endourol. 2008;22:1709–13.

Malik SA, Ahmad Z, Shumaila S, Javaid G. Hydatid cyst of the kidney. Biomedica. 2007;23:60–2.

Mongha R, Narayan S, Kundu AK. Primary hydatid cyst of kidney and ureter with gross hydatiduria: A case report and evaluation of radiological features. Indian J Urol. 2008;24:116–7.

Ozden E, Bostanci Y, Mercimek MN, Yakupoglu YK, Yilmaz AF, Sarıkaya S. Renal hydatid cyst treatment: retroperitoneoscopic "closed cyst" pericystectomy. Int J Urol. 2011;18:237–9.

Pinar P, Mecit K, Fatih A, Selami S, Melike BK, Adnan O. Hydatid disease from head to toe. Radiographics. 2003;23:475–94.

Poulios C. Echinococcal disease of urinary tract: review of management of 7 cases. J Urol. 1991;145:924–7.

Prabhudessai SC, Patankar RV, Bradoo A. Laparoscopic treatment of renal hydatid cyst. J Minim Access Surg. 2009;5:20–1.

Rami R, Khattala K, ElMadi A, Afifi MA, Bouabddallah Y. The renal hydatid cyst: report on 4 cases. Pan Afr Med J. 2011;8:31.

Reddy CR, Narasiah IL, Parvathi G, Rao MS. Epidemiology of hydatid disease in Kurnool. Indian J Med Res. 1968;56:1205–20.

Shah KJ, Ganpule AP, Desai MR. Isolated renal hydatid cyst managed by laparoscopic transperitoneal nephrectomy. Indian J Urol. 2009;25:531–3.

Shukla A, Garge S, Verma P. A case of large renal hydatid cyst. Saudi J Kidney Dis Transpl. 2011;22:538–40.

Tryfonas GJ, Avtzoglou PP, Chaidos C, Zioutis J, Gavopoulos S, Limas C. Renal hydatid disease: diagnosis and treatment. J Pediatr Surg. 1993;28:228–31.

Von Lictenberg F, Lehman JS. Parasitic diseases of the genitourinary system. In: Harrison JH, Gittes RF, Perlmutter AD, Stamey TA, Walsh PC, editors. Campbell's urology, vol. 1. 4th ed. Philadelphia, PA: Saunders; 1978. p. 631–3.

Primary Extrahepatic Abdominal Hydatidosis

Hydatid disease in humans also known as echinococcosis is caused by four known species of *Echinococcus*, namely, *Echinococcus granulosus*, *E. multilocularis*, *E. vogeli* and *E. oligarthus*. Only the former three are of medical importance. *E. granulosus* causes cystic hydatid disease, whereas *E. multilocularis* causes alveolar hydatid disease. *E. multilocularis* is rare and the most virulent, while *E. vogeli* is the rarest variant.

Etiology

Echinococcus belongs to the phylum Platyhelminthes (tapeworms). The life cycle of echinococcus involves two hosts which include one definitive host such as wolf, foxes, hyenas, jackals and dogs and the other intermediate host which include grass grazing animals such as sheep, cattle, goats, horses and some other animals. Humans act as an accidental intermediate host.

The adult worm lives in the small gut of definitive host and releases thousands of eggs which are passed to the exterior along with faeces. Metacestode develops within these eggs outside. These embryonated eggs are ingested by intermediate host or humans along with contaminated grass, vegetables or water. Egg shell is dissolved, and larvae are released which enter into the portal circulation and from there are carried anywhere to the body and infest the liver, lungs, muscles and other organs.

Pathophysiology

Once the contaminated food is taken by humans, hexacanth embryos reach the liver via portal circulation. As a result, majority of the hydatid cysts develop in the liver. However some hexacanths escape the hepatic filter and reach to the lungs after passing through the heart. Extrahepatic extrapulmonary hydatid occurs in those cases

© Springer Nature Singapore Pte Ltd. 2019
A. A. Malik, S. Bari, *Human Abdominal Hydatidosis*,
https://doi.org/10.1007/978-981-13-2152-8_9

where these return to the heart from lungs and then enter the systemic circulation leading to dissemination to other extrahepatic extrapulmonary organs (Engin et al. 2000). Extrahepatic involvement may occur directly following lymphatic spread from the gut into the systemic circulation (Morris and Richards 1992; Makni et al. 2013).

Epidemiology

Echinococcosis remains an endemic disease in Mediterranean countries, the Middle East, Central Asia China, the southern part of South America, Iceland, Australia, New Zealand and southern parts of Africa (Orhan et al. 2003). Both the sexes are equally involved. The cysts grow slowly. Although any age group may be involved, cystic echinococcosis usually involves younger adults mostly between 30 and 40 years, whereas alveolar echinococcosis is seen in elderly patients usually above 50 years.

Signs and Symptoms

More than 70% of the patients are asymptomatic, even into advanced age. The symptomology is usually determined by the parasite the size of the cyst and location of the cysts and severity of the infection. Patients usually give history of living in or visiting an endemic area. It is important to establish history of exposure to the parasite. Patients may give history of ingestion of contaminated foods or water. Primary and isolated extrahepatic intra-abdominal hydatid cysts (PIEHC) are rare (Hamamci et al. 2004).

Hydatid Disease of the Spleen

Although hydatid disease of the spleen is rare, the spleen is the commonest organ involved after the liver and lungs and forms less than 2% of total cases of hydatid disease (Ozdogan et al. 2001). The spleen is involved either due to spread of disease via bloodstream or following intra-abdominal rupture of hydatid liver cysts and is usually solitary. The splenic hydatid has all the radiologic features typical of hydatid. The differential diagnosis of splenic hydatidosis includes pseudocysts, splenic abscess, hematoma and rarely splenic tumour (Dede et al. 2002; Wani et al. 2005; Dar et al. 2002).

Peritoneal Hydatid Disease

Peritoneal hydatidosis is usually secondary to intra-abdominal rupture of hepatic hydatid or may develop after surgery for hydatid due to spillage. However primary peritoneal hydatidosis has been reported. Although it is usually asymptomatic,

Fig. 1 CT image primary
extrahepatic multiple
unilocular hydatid cysts

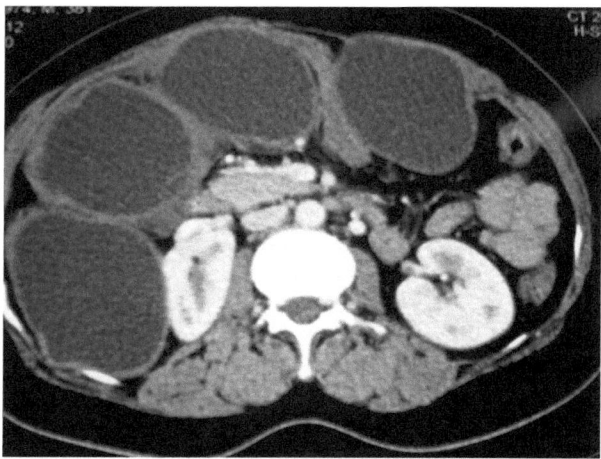

Fig. 2 CT image of
primary peritoneal
multilocular hydatid cyst

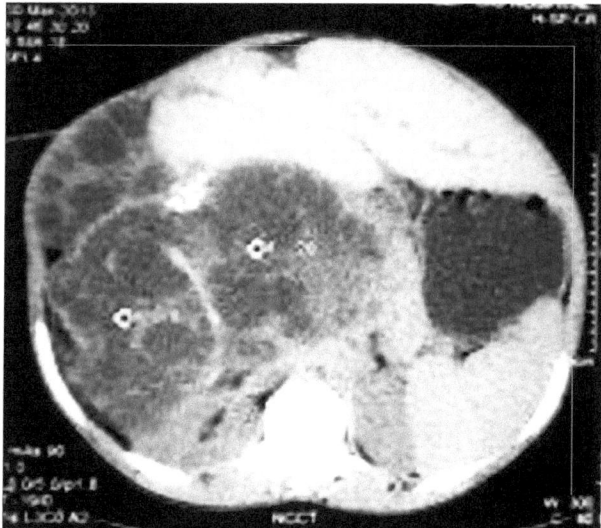

abdominal distension, mass per abdomen or compression symptoms leading to urinary retention may be present in some patients (Daali et al. 2000). CT Abdomen is
the investigation of choice for diagnosis of primary extrahepatic abdominal hydatidosis. CT scan shows a multi-cystic pelvic-abdominal mass with a smooth outer
cyst wall, with or without specks and calcification (Figs. 1 and 2).

Hydatid Disease of Adrenals

Hydatid cysts of the adrenal gland are also rare even in areas where the disease is
endemic (Horchani et al. 2006). In more than 90% cases adrenal hydatid is unilat-
eral. Patients usually remain asymptomatic for years together and are diagnosed

accidently when patients are exposed to radiological work for some other disease. Very few patients may become symptomatic depending on the size, site and number of cysts and their relation to adjacent organs. Some patients may present once a complication develops such as pressure effect on surrounding organs such as renal artery resulting into arterial hypertension or fistula formation. In early stages it looks like a simple cysts. However mature cyst will have daughter cysts and floating membranes in with some calcification. Nonparasitic cysts such as endothelial cysts, pseudocysts and epithelial cysts need to be differentiated (Habib et al. 2002).

Hydatid Disease of the Pancreas

Hydatid disease of the pancreas is exceptional, and its incidence ranges from 0.14 to 2%. Clinical features depend on the size and location of the cysts in pancreas (Brown et al. 1995). Although cysts located in the distal part of the pancreas such as tail and body are usually asymptomatic (Suryawanshi et al. 2011), few patients may present with abdominal swelling with subsequent pressure symptoms. A cyst located in the head of pancreas may cause compression of CBD resulting into obstructive jaundice. Rarely, patients with pancreatic hydatid can also present with acute pancreatitis. As the preoperative diagnosis of primary pancreatic hydatid cyst is difficult, high index of suspicion is necessary. Radiological imaging is mandatory for diagnosis. Surgery is the treatment of choice for managing pancreatic hydatid disease and includes central pancreatectomy, distal pancreatectomy or pancreato-duodenectomy depending upon the location of the cyst. Hydatid cyst pancreas can also drained percutaneously using hypertonic (20%) saline as a scolicidal agent. Haemorrhage and pancreatic fistula are the major complications of surgical resection (Dede et al. 2002; Wani et al. 2005).

Hydatid Disease of the Kidney

Hydatid disease of the kidney is extremely rare and constitutes only 2–3% of all cases. Most patients with renal hydatid disease are between 30 and 50 years of age (Buckley et al. 1985). The cyst is usually single and lies in the cortex of the kidney (Buckley et al. 1985). Patients may be asymptomatic if the cyst is closed and not communicating with the pelvis. The cyst may achieve a huge size before becoming symptomatic, and symptoms may vary according to the size and extent of the cyst. A mass palpable in the lumber area is the only clinical sign (Buckley et al. 1985). Symptomatic patients may present with lumbar pain, haematuria, intermittent fever or hypertension.

Hydatiduria is a pathognomonic feature renal hydatid disease although, macroscopic hydatiduria is rarely documented. Microscopic hydatiduria may be seen in 10–20% of cases of renal hydatidosis (Kiresi et al. 2003). It is characterized by an episode of renal colic followed by passage of grapelike material in the urine. The specific diagnosis of hydatid disease is based on identifying protoscoleces or hooklets in cyst fluid, but usually fluid aspiration is not recommended due to risk of fluid leakage and anaphylaxis reaction (Reddy et al. 1968). Saline mount, modified

Baxby staining procedure and haematoxylin and eosin staining can be done on cyst fluid for better visualization of hooklets.

Pelvic Hydatid Disease

Pelvis is as an uncommon site for hydatid cyst and is involved in 0.3–4.27% of cases. Preoperative diagnosis of pelvic hydatid is very difficult and poses a diagnostic problem (Dirican et al. 2008). Hydatid disease of the female genital tract is extremely rare and usually develops after intra-abdominal rupture of hydatid liver or due to spillage during surgery for primary disease of the some other abdominal organs. Although the exact mechanism of primary pelvic involvement is not known, it is believed that scoleces reach the pelvis through the lymphatics or bloodstream (Uchikova et al. 2009).

The ovary is the most common genital organs involved and constitutes 0.2% of all the cases of hydatid disease locations (Aksu et al. 1997; Baba et al. 1991; Bellil et al. 2009). In those cases where the uterus has been affected, hydatid vesicles may be encountered during vaginal examination (Gueddana et al. 1990). Patients with pelvic hydatid are usually asymptomatic, or they may have a non-specific presentation. Some patients may present chronic pelvic pain and abdominal swelling (Hangval et al. 1979; Gamoudi et al. 1995). Others may present with infertility and irregular menstrual cycle. Immunological tests have got very low sensitivity and specificity in case of pelvic hydatid disease and there is a very high a risk of false negatives cases. Eosinophilia may be seen in around 30% of cases. Ultrasound is the cheapest modality for diagnosis of the disease. It is the method of choice with high specificity (Diaz-Recasens et al. 1998). However, complicated ovarian cysts may be difficult to differentiate from ovarian malignancy on imaging. CT scan has got a high sensitivity and is a method of choice for diagnosis (Fig. 3). MRI is considered as useful investigation to classify cysts with high specificity and is quite valuable for differentiating pelvic hydatid from certain benign tumours such as myxoid tumours and myxoid neurofibroma. Chest radiograph helps us to rule out any concomitant pulmonary hydatid cyst (Varedi et al. 2008).

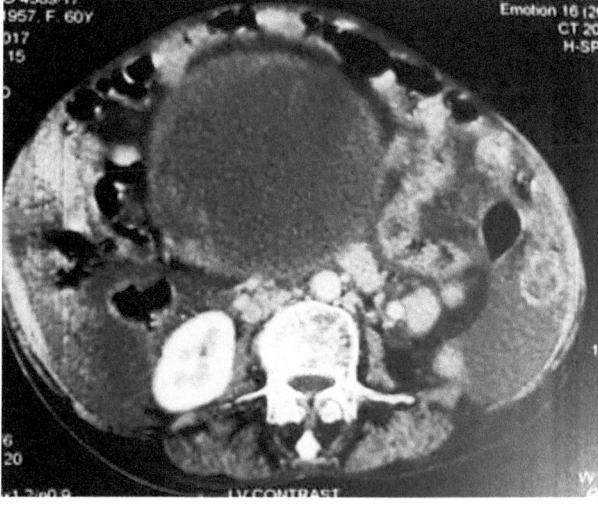

Fig. 3 Primary extrahepatic pelvic hydatid seen on CT image

Treatment

Complete surgical excision of the intact cyst (cysto-pericystectomy) (Figs. 4 and 5) is the treatment of choice (Durgun et al. 2003; Suryawanshi et al. 2011). Care has to be taken to avoid leakage of cyst content that can cause anaphylactic reaction and recurrence. It may also lead to the dissemination of the disease. If the cysto-pericystectomy is impossible, enucleation of the cyst has to be carried out (Fig. 6) in which the cyst contents (fluid, membrane and daughter cysts) are removed intra-operatively after isolating the operative area, and the cyst pouch has to be flushed with any of the available scolicidal solutions (Bickers 1970). Scolicidal solutions need to be kept in the cavity for a sufficient amount of time for full scolicidal action depending upon the nature of the agent. Other options include percutaneous drain-age of the cyst under ultrasound guidance (PAIR). In this technique needle aspira-tion of cyst contents is done followed by irrigation of scolicidal solutions and then

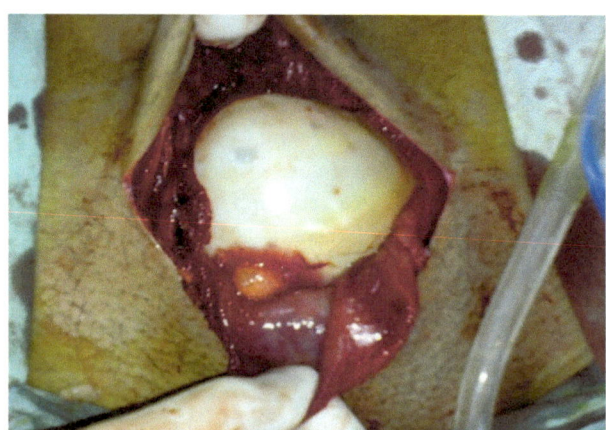

Fig. 4 Intraoperative view of extrahepatic primary peritoneal hydatid cyst

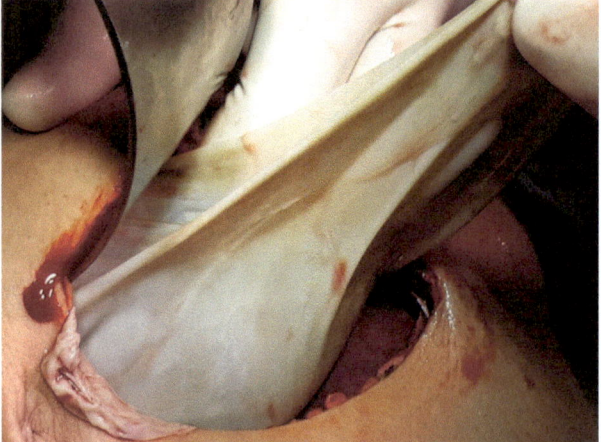

Fig. 5 Primary extrahepatic peritoneal hydatid cyst being delivered

Fig. 6 Classical hydatid cyst and membrane

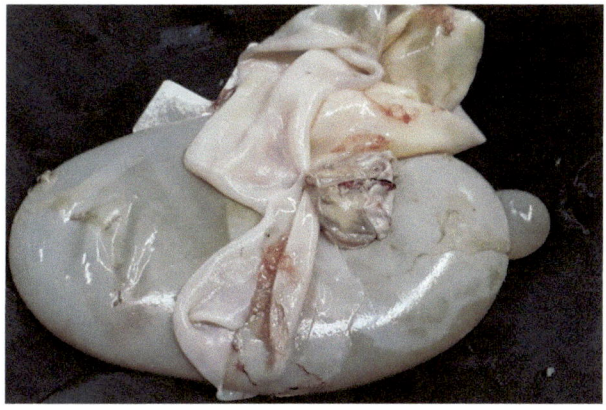

reaspiration. Medical management using albendazole therapy is another option available (Yattoo et al. 1999). Albendazole therapy may be given preoperatively and then continued postoperatively or may be started after surgery only depending upon whether diagnosis was available before surgery.

Complications

Complications usually encountered include infection of the cyst, distortion or loss of function of affected organs and pressure effect on adjacent organs (Akbulut et al. 2010). Rupture of the echinococcal cyst may occur leading to anaphylaxis and widespread dissemination or secondary echinococosis and recurrence after treatment. Complications related to surgery and drugs used during anaesthesia can also be seen. Medical therapy can also lead to drug-induced toxicity like hepatotoxicity, anaemia, thrombocytopenia, alopecia and teratogenicity.

Complications can also develop during percutaneous aspiration such as bleeding, trauma to adjacent organs, infections, allergic reaction or anaphylaxis. In some cases, aspiration may be incomplete, and some daughter cysts may persist in the mother cyst leading to recurrence, while in other cases, sudden decompression of the cyst can occur resulting in biliary fistulas. Lately, chemical sclerosing cholangitis may develop in those patients where scolicidal agents were used.

References

Akbulut S, Senol A, Ekin A, Bakir S, Bayan K, et al. Primary retroperitoneal hydatid cyst: report of 2 cases and review of 41 published cases. Int Surg. 2010;95:189–96.

Aksu MF, Budak E, Ince U, Aksu C. Hydatid cyst of the ovary. Arch Gynecol Obstet. 1997;261:51–3.

Baba A, Chaieb A, Khairi H, Keskes J. Epidemiological profile of pelvic hydatidosis: 15 cases [in French]. J Gynecol Obstet Biol Reprod (Paris). 1991;20:657–60.

Bellil S, Limaiem F, Bellil K, Chelly I, Mekni A, et al. Epidemiology of extra pulmonary hydatid cysts: 265 Tunisian cases. Med Mal Infect. 2009;39:341–3.

Bickers WM. Hydatid disease of the female pelvis. Amer J Obstet Gynaecol. 1970;107:477–83.

Brown RA, Millar AJ, Steiner Z, Krige JE, Burkimsher D, Cywes S. Hydatid cyst of the pancreas. A case report in a child. Eur J Pediatr Surg. 1995;5:121–3.

Buckley RJ, Smith S, Herschorn S, et al. Echinococcal disease of the kidney presenting as a renal filling defect. J Urol. 1985;133:660–1.

Daali M, Hssaida R, Zoubir M, et al. Peritoneal hydatidosis: a study of 25 cases in Morocco. Sante. 2000;10(4):255–60.

Dar MA, Shah OJ, Wani NA, et al. Surgical management of splenic hydatidosis. Surg Today. 2002;32(3):224–9.

Dede S, Dede H, Caliskan E, Demir B. Recurrent pelvic hydatid cyst obstructing labor, with a concomitant hepatic primary: a case report. J Reprod Med. 2002;47:164–6.

Diaz-Recasens J, Garcia-Enguidanos A, Munoz I, Sainz de la Cuesta R. Ultrasonographic appearance of an Echinococcus ovarian cyst. Obstet Gynecol. 1998;1998(91):841–2.

Dirican A, Unal B, Kayaalp C, Kirimlioglu V. Subcutaneous hydatid cysts occurring in the palm and the thigh: two case reports. J Med Case Rep. 2008;13:273.

Durgun V, Kapan S, Kapan M, et al. Primary splenic hydatidosis. Dig Surg. 2003;20(1):38–41.

Engin G, Acunas B, Rozanes I, et al. Hydatid disease with unusual localization. Eur Radiol. 2000;10:1904–12.

Gamoudi A, Ben Romdhane K, Farhat K, Khattech R, Hechiche M, et al. Ovarian hydatic cyst: 7 cases [in French]. J Gynecol Obstet Biol Reprod (Paris). 1995;24:144–8.

Gueddana F, Chemmen-Lebbene L, Lebbi I, et al. Intrauterine hydatidosis. A case report. J Gynecol Obstet Biol Reprod (Paris). 1990;19:725–7.

Habib RM, Khan R, Harris SH. Hydatid cyst of gallbladder. Ind J Gastroenterol. 2002;22(2):67–8.

Hamamci EO, Besim H, Korkmaz A. Unusual locations of the hydatid disease and surgical approach. ANZ J Surg. 2004;74:356–60.

Hangval H, Habibi H, Moshref A, Rahimi A. Case report of an ovarian hydatid cyst. J Trop Med Hyg. 1979;82:34.

Horchani A, Nouira Y, Nouira K, et al. Hydatid cyst of the adrenal gland: a clinical study of six cases. Sci World J. 2006;6:2420–5.

Kiresi DA, Karabacakoglu A, Odev K, Karaköse S. Uncommon locations of hydatid cysts. Acta Radiol. 2003;2003(44):622–36.

Makni A, Jouini M, Kacem M, et al. Extra-hepatic intra-abdominal hydatid cyst: which characteristic, compared to the hepatic location? Updates Surg. 2013;65(1):25–33.

Morris DL, Richards KS. Biology of Echinococcus. Hydatid disease. Current medical and surgical management. Oxford: Butterworth Heinemann; 1992. p. 7.

Orhan Z, Kara H, Tuzuner T, Sencan I, Alper M. Primary subcutaneous cyst hydatic disease in proximal thigh: an unusual localisation: a case report. BMC Musculoskelet Disord. 2003; 7:25.

Ozdogan M, Baykal A, Keskek M, et al. Hydatid cyst of the spleen: treatment options. Int Surg. 2001;86(2):122–6.

Reddy CR, Narasiah IL, Parvathi G, Rao MS. Epidemiology of hydatid disease in Kurnool. Indian J Med Res. 1968;56:1205–20. [PubMed]

Suryawanshi P, Khan AQ, Jatal S. Primary hydatid cyst of pancreas with acute pancreatitis. Int J Surg Case Rep. 2011;2:122–4.

Uchikova E, Pehlivanov B, Uchikov A, Shipkov C, Poriazova EA. Primary ovarian hydatid cyst. Aust N Z J Obstet Gynaecol. 2009;49:441–2.

Varedi P, Saadat Mostafavi SR, Salouti R, Saedi D, Nabavizadeh SA, et al. Hydatidosis of the pelvic cavity: a big masquerade. Infect Dis Obstet Gynecol. 2008;2008:782621.

Wani RA, Malik AA, Chowdri NA, et al. Primary extrahepatic abdominal hydatidosis. Int J Surg. 2005;3:125–7.

Yattoo GN, Khuroo MS, Zargar SA, Bhat FA, Sofi BA. Case report: percutaneous drainage of the pancreatic head hydatid cyst with obstructive jaundice. J Gastroenterol Hepatol. 1999;14: 931–4.

Minimally Invasive Management of Hepatic Hydatidosis

Hydatid disease is a worldwide parasitic disease that is endemic in certain parts of the world, such as Australia, New Zealand, Mediterranean countries, Turkey, North Africa, South America, the Philippines, Northern China, and the Indian subcontinent (Buttenschoen and Carli Buttenschoen 2003).

Human hydatidosis is caused by the larval form of the tapeworm genus Echinococcus, which belongs to the family Taenidae. Four species of Echinococcus cause disease in humans (Milicevic 2002; Christian and Pitt 2007). *Echinococcus granulosus* and *E. multilocularis* are the most common, causing cystic echinococcosis and alveolar echinococcosis, respectively. The two other species, *E. Vogeli* and *E. oligarthus*, cause polycystic echinococcosis, but have rarely been associated with human infection. Besides these four, two new species have been identified: *E. shiquicus*, isolated from small mammals in the Tibetan plateau, and *E. felidis* in African lions; however, their potential to transmit the disease is not known.

The adult *E. granulosus* resides in the small bowel of the definitive hosts, dogs or other canines. Gravid proglottids release eggs in the intestines of the definitive host that are passed in the feces. After the ingestion of tainted herbage by a suitable intermediate host (under natural conditions: sheep, cattle, camels, goats, horses), the egg hatches in the small bowel and releases an oncosphere (Milicevic 2002). This penetrates the intestinal wall and migrates through the circulatory system into various organs, especially the liver and lungs. In these organs, the oncosphere develops into a cyst that enlarges gradually, producing daughter cysts that fill the cyst interior. The cycle is completed when dogs eat the cyst-bearing organs of the intermediate host. Humans are inadvertent intermediate hosts who become infected by consuming contaminated unwashed vegetables and by contact with infected animals or contaminated soil (Bilge and Sozuer 1994).

Patients may be completely asymptomatic or may have non-specific symptoms, such as pain in the right upper quadrant or in the epigastrium, depending on the cyst's site, size, stage of development, and viability and whether the cyst is infected (Milicevic 2002). Some patients may present with fever, fatigue, and nausea, and

© Springer Nature Singapore Pte Ltd. 2019
A. A. Malik, S. Bari, *Human Abdominal Hydatidosis*,
https://doi.org/10.1007/978-981-13-2152-8_10

dyspepsia may also be present. A right palpable mass or hepatomegaly is the most common sign.

Routine laboratory tests give variable results and have no specific role in diagnosis (Sayek 2004). Serological tests help in screening as well as in diagnosis of the disease. Chest radiographs or abdominal radiographs may show an elevated dome of the diaphragm or a calcified rim. Ultrasonography (US) and computed tomography (CT) are the main diagnostic tools for the detection of hydatid disease (Sayek 2004; Bari et al. 2011). CT of the abdomen is more informative as far as the size, location, and number of cysts is concerned. Although magnetic resonance imaging provides better structural details, it is less cost-effective than US or CT scans (Balik et al. 1999). Endoscopic retrograde cholangiopancreatography (ERCP) has a role in patients where cysto-biliary communication is suspected (Sayek 2004).

There is still much debate about the management of liver hydatidosis (Zaharie and Bartos 2013; Busic et al. 2012). The objective of managing hydatid disease is to completely eradicate the parasite and prevent any future recurrence. Various factors determine the treatment modality for uncomplicated hydatid disease; these include the health status of the patient; the number, size, and location of the cysts; and the presence of any complications. Originally, open surgery was the main acknowledged treatment for this disease. In recent times, however, many changes in modality have occurred, starting with echo-guided puncture, which met with strong opposition, as it contradicted all the principles of hydatid surgery, particularly that of puncturing the cyst without the fear of spillage of the hydatid fluid (Mamarajabov et al. 2011).

There are three main modalities of treatment for hydatid cyst of the liver: chemotherapy, surgery, and minimally invasive procedures. Minimally invasive procedures include the puncture, aspiration, injection, reaspiration (PAIR technique), ERCP, and the laparoscopic approach. Minimally invasive techniques have well documented advantages that have increased their utility in recent times. Khoury et al. (1994) was the first to perform percutaneous aspiration, while Saglam (1996) was the first to perform laparoscopic drainage (Saglam 1996). Bickel et al. (1994), in their study, reported ten cases of hydatid cyst managed laparoscopically. There was no mortality or relapse in any of the patients. Another 16 cases of hydatid cyst were managed laparoscopically by Alper et al. (1995); 4 of these patients developed postoperative abscesses, but there was no relapse.

Percutaneous Aspiration, Injection, and Reaspiration (PAIR)

PAIR is a newer minimally invasive procedure that involves percutaneous aspiration of the cyst contents under US guidance, followed by the introduction of a proto scolicidal agent into the cyst, and finally re-aspiration of the contents, thus completing the procedure (Sayek 2004). This results in the miniaturization of the cyst, in both size and volume, and thickening of the cyst wall, which also becomes irregular. The fluid component of the cyst decreases and the cyst finally solidifies (Sayek 2004). On US, this solid remnant looks like a pseudotumor. Khuroo et al. (1997) conducted a control study comparing cystectomy with percutaneous aspiration and found that the minimally invasive approach was associated with a shorter hospital stay.

Modifications of the PAIR technique, such as PAIR catheterization, have also been employed. The PAIR method and its indications have recently been revised under the supervision of the World Health Organization (WHO/OIE 2001). Contraindications of the procedure include an uncooperative or younger patient (less than 3 years of age), complicated cysts, inaccessible cysts, and cysts in risky locations.

Endoscopic Retrograde Cholangiopancreatography

Endoscopic retrograde cholangiopancreatography (ERCP) can be used as a diagnostic as well as a therapeutic modality in the management of complicated hydatid cyst of the liver. Preoperatively, ERCP helps to delineate complications related to the biliary tract, to assess and manage acute conditions such as biliary obstruction and cholangitis, so that an elective procedure can be performed later. In cases of frank biliary rupture, ERCP can help in clearing out the common bile duct (CBD), thereby avoiding the need to explore the CBD later in the course of elective treatment (Fig. 1). Postoperatively, ERCP has, again, a significant role in the examination of the entire biliary tract, along with any distortion in anatomy, as may happen in recurrent cases; this modality also helps in the endoscopic management of biliary fistula and strictures (Sayek 2004).

Laparoscopic Hydatid Liver Surgery

The laparoscopic approach to hepatic hydatid cyst was introduced in 1993 as an alternative to the classic open surgery (Ertem and Karahasanoglu 2002; Gupta et al. 2014). As is done in open surgery, complete removal of the cyst, evacuation of its contents, deroofing, and obliteration of the cyst cavity can be carried out very easily (Alper et al. 1995; Saglam 1996). The laparoscopic approach has its own

Fig. 1 Endoscopic sphincterotomy performed in a patient with persistent postoperative biliary leak communication from the cavity of a hydatid cyst in the liver

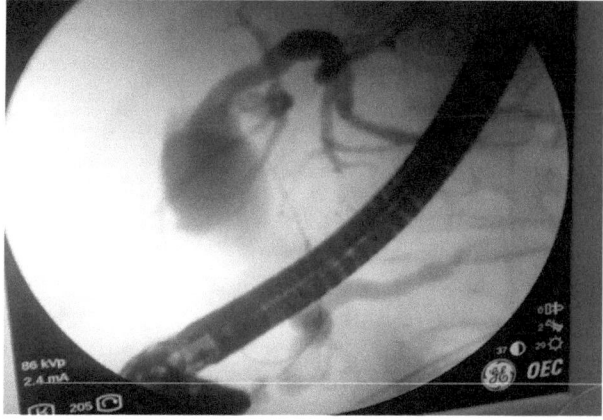

Fig. 2 Type 1 hydatid cyst
in the right lobe of the liver
managed laparoscopically

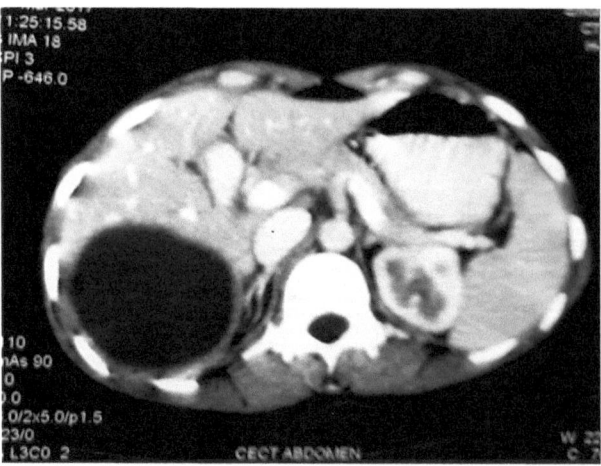

advantages and disadvantages, with the advantages being the ability to carry out detailed examination of the cyst cavity; its minimally invasive nature; a shorter hospital stay for the patient; and fewer wound-related complications (Rihani et al. 2005; Rooh-ul-Muqim et al. 2011; Sayek and Onat 2001). On the downside, the laparoscopic approach is less feasible in complicated cysts and in difficult locations, and there is a risk of spillage and seeding (Fig. 2). All the principles of open surgery are also applied to the laparoscopic approach (Bickel et al. 1994; Bickel and Eitan 1995; Bhadreshwara et al. 2015).

Surgical Technique

After the patient has been draped, the first step is to create a pneumoperitoneum via a supra-umbilical port (Malik et al. 2017). The next step is to introduce a 10-mm port through the same supra-umbilical incision. This is followed by inspection of the whole abdominal cavity to look for cysts in places other than the liver, or any other finding. Two more ports are placed: a 12-mm port in the epigastric area 5 cm below the xiphisternum and a 5-mm port in the right subcostal area in the anterior axillary line between the epigastric and umbilical ports (Fig. 3). After the cyst has been identified, two gauze packs soaked in a scolicidal agent are pushed into the abdominal cavity through the 10-mm port (Malik et al. 2017). These two packs are placed around the cyst to take care of any spillage that may occur during surgery (Fig. 4). An aspiration needle is introduced through the epigastric port to aspirate the cyst contents, and a suction cannula is introduced through the subcostal port to suck out any fluid that may spill while the cyst contents are aspirated; around 60–70% of the hydatid fluid is sucked out. If the cyst contents are not bile-stained, the scolicidal agent is injected into cyst, where it remains for 10–15 min. After 10–15 min, suction is done again and the cyst contents are again sucked out (Fig. 5). Up to this

Fig. 3 Port position in laparoscopic hydatid surgery

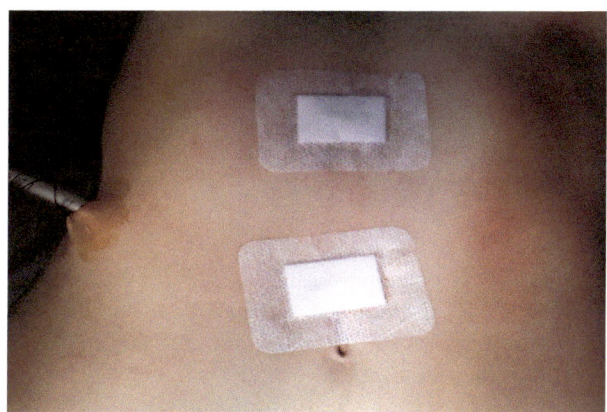

Fig. 4 Hydatid cyst in left lobe of liver as seen on laparoscopy

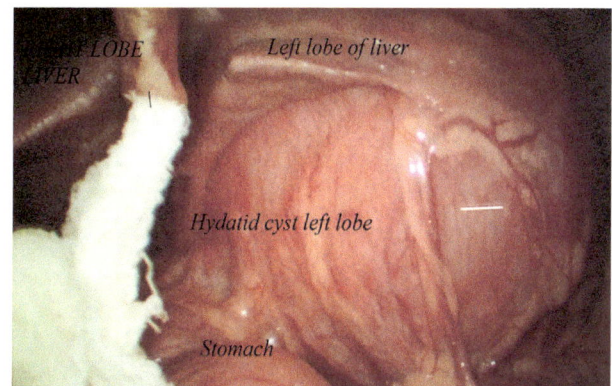

Fig. 5 Hydatid cyst in right lobe of liver being aspirated with a suction cannula inside the cavity

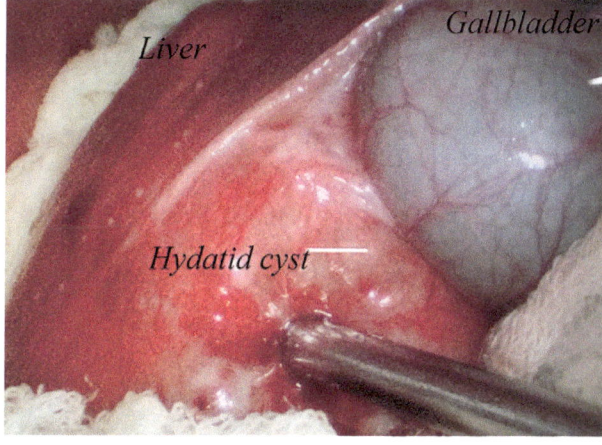

time, only the fluid contents have been sucked out and the solid contents are still in the cyst cavity. For removing solid contents such as membranes and daughter cysts, the cyst wall is opened using thermal cautery, which is introduced through the epigastric port, while a suction cannula is introduced through a subcostal port and the residual contents are sucked out. The laminated membrane and daughter cysts, if any, are collected into a sterile bag, which is placed in the abdominal cavity. Once all the cyst contents are collected in the bag, it is delivered outside (Fig. 6). After this the laparoscopic camera is introduced into the cyst cavity to rule out any major cysto-biliary communication and any side wall cysts (Fig. 7). The residual cyst cavity is again examined. Finally the omentum is placed inside the abdominal cavity and a suture or clip is applied to hold the omentum. In our clinical practice we routinely place a drain in the abdominal cavity as well (Malik et al. 2017). The port sites are sutured and antiseptic dressings are applied.

Fig. 6 Laminated membrane being delivered during laparoscopic hydatid cystectomy

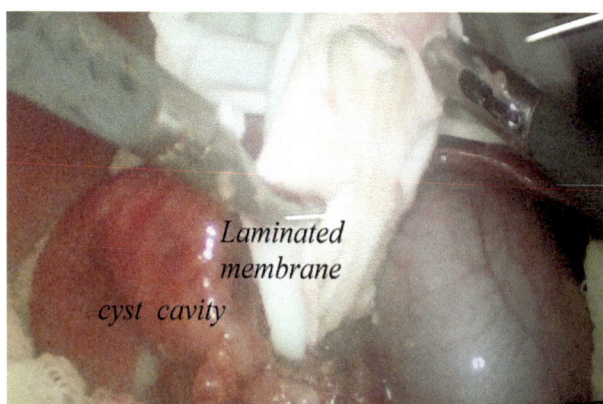

Fig. 7 Inner side of the cyst cavity as seen with a laparoscope placed into the cavity

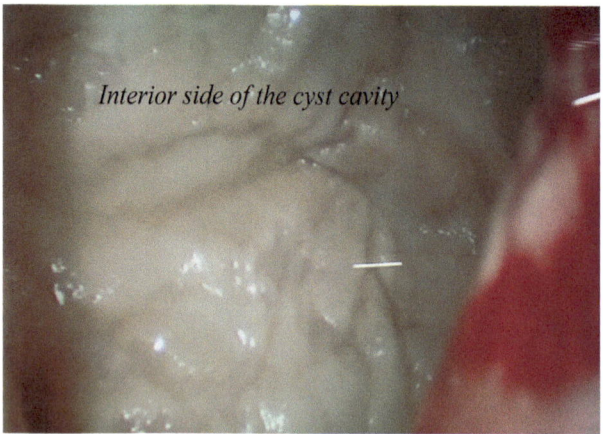

Fig. 8 Palanivelu hydatid
system

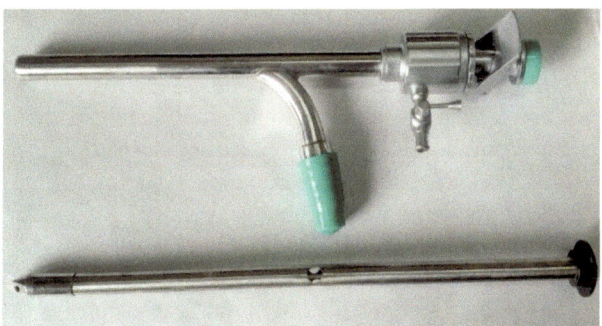

The Palanivelu Hydatid System (PHS)

The components of the PHS include a trocar, cannula, and two reducers, one of which is 5 mm and the other is 3 mm (Fig. 8). The length of the trocar is 29 cm. The trocar is hollow throughout its length so that it can accommodate a suction cannula. The tip of the trocar is in the shape of a pyramid and each facet of the pyramid has a hole, so that if there is any leakage of any fluid during its insertion, the fluid is sucked into the trocar's hollow body by the cannula placed within it. The trocar's shaft has two holes, which are placed opposite each other at a distance of 17 cm from the tip. The length of the cannula is 26 cm and it has an internal diameter of 12 mm. The cannula has two side channels, one for the insufflation of gas and the other for suction. The inner diameter of the suction channel is 10 mm. The shape and design of the outer nozzle is such that the suction tubing fits onto it in an airtight manner.

Laparoscopic Surgery Technique Using the Palanivelu Hydatid System

A pneumoperitoneum is created as usual through the umbilicus and a camera port is introduced through the same opening. The laparoscope is introduced through the camera port and the hydatid cyst is identified and localized. This is followed by the introduction of the PHS trocar into the peritoneal cavity directly over the area harboring the hydatid cyst (Jauhari and Golhar 2014). Once the PHS is within the abdominal cavity, the trocar is removed and only the cannula is advanced toward the liver surface, until the tip of the cannula comes into close contact with the exposed surface of the hydatid cyst. Once the cannula is in close contact with the cyst surface, suction is applied through the side channel so that there is airtight contact between the surface of the cyst and the opening of the cannula. After this we again introduce a trocar with a 5-mm suction nozzle inside it into the cannula. This suction nozzle is connected to another suction machine. Steady pressure is applied and the trocar is pushed into the cyst, along with the cannula. While puncturing the cyst wall, if there is any spillage of fluid, the fluid is immediately sucked up either into the body of the hollow trocar through its fenestrated tip and then into the suction cannula or into the outer cannula and then into the suction side-channel (Jauhari and Golhar 2014). Once the PHS is inside the hydatid cyst, the trocar is removed, the suction nozzle is reintroduced thorough the main channel, and thorough irrigation is carried out; at the same time, continuous suction is simultaneously maintained all along ? to suck out the cyst contents. With the help of PHS, it is easy to remove all the cyst contents, which include fragments of the laminated membrane, daughter cysts, and debris (Jauhari and Golhar 2014).

After the cyst contents have been evacuated, CO_2 insufflation is reduced to a pressure of 3 mmHg–4 mmHg and a telescope is introduced into the cyst cavity through the cannula to inspect the interior of the cyst cavity for any daughter cyst or membranes left behind and to inspect for any overt biliary leak (Fig. 7). Once overt cysto-biliary communication is ruled out, either by the absence of bile staining in the evacuated fluid or by non-visualization of any bile leak within the cyst cavity (Jauhari and Golhar 2014), scolicidal agents have to be instilled into the cyst cavity. Although a number of scolicidal agents are available and any of them can be used depending on the surgeon's choice, cetrimide 0.5% is the most commonly used scolicidal agent used in laparoscopic hydatid surgery (Hanan 2005).The scolicidal agent is kept within the cavity for at least 10–15 min to be effective. After 10–15 min, the scolicidal agent is sucked out and the residual cavity is dealt with by any of the standard methods. In our surgical practice we either do a marsupialization of the residual cavity if the cyst is small and superficial or we place an external tube drain into the cavity, either alone or along with omentopexy if the cavity is large and deep. If there are signs of cysto-biliary communication, the use of a scolicidal agent is avoided. Cysto-biliary communications are identified and closed using 3-0 Vicryl. This is followed by omentoplasty and external tube drainage of the cavity. In addition to this, another tube drain is always placed outside the cavity in all cases.

Clinical Studies

In recent times several studies have been conducted to compare the results of open surgery with those of laparoscopic surgery for hydatid disease of the liver (Bickel et al. 2001; Baskaran and Patnaik 2004). Bickel et al. (2001) conducted laparoscopic surgery in 31 consecutive patients with hydatid liver disease, with no selection criteria. The median follow-up period was 49 months and there were no recurrences. The authors came to the conclusion that the laparoscopic approach could be used safely in all abdominal hydatid cysts.

The present authors also conducted a study comparing laparoscopic surgery with conventional surgery for hepatic hydatid disease (Malik et al. 2017). The study population comprised 80 patients; 40 had laparoscopic surgery and 40 had open surgery. All the patients were adults, with the cysts located in liver segments 3, 4, 5, 6, and 8, with no evidence of calcifications, major biliary communication, or cyst infection. Patients with cysts located in segments 1, 2, and 7 of the liver and those with multiple liver hydatid cysts or cysts located near vascular liver elements were not included in the study (Malik et al. 2017). Patients with deep-seated cysts, recurrent cysts, or ruptured hydatid cysts, and patients with severe cardio-pulmonary compromise and previous multiple upper abdominal surgeries were also excluded from the study.

The patients in the two groups were statistically comparable in regard to age distribution and sex ratio. More than 55% of the patients presented with abdominal pain, while 15% of the patients had an abdominal mass (Malik et al. 2017). In both the laparoscopic and open groups, most of the patients had a single univesicular cyst located in the right lobe of the liver. In the laparoscopic group, biliary leak was the most common complication (7.50%); it was treated conservatively and resolved spontaneously after 3–4 days. On the other hand, in patients managed by the open surgical method, surgical site infection was the commonest complication (10%).

The average operative time for the laparoscopic group was 89.80 min (range, 60–120 min), while the average operative time was only 60.43 min (40–80 min) for open surgery. Two of the 40 patients who underwent laparoscopic surgery had to be converted to open surgery (Malik et al. 2017). In the laparoscopic group, hospital stay varied from 2 to 6 days, while hospital stay was 5–12 days in the open group. In the laparoscopic group the patients returned to their routine work within 8.10 days (range, 6–12 days); in comparison, the patients who underwent open surgery took 20.70 days (range, 10–25 days) to return to normal routine work. None of the patients in the laparoscopic group had a recurrence, while recurrence was seen in 2 (5%) patients who underwent open surgery (Malik et al. 2017).

Based on results from various studies we can conclude that laparoscopic hydatid surgery is safe and feasible in selected patients, the main advantages being the lower postoperative morbidity, and recurrence rate.

Limitations of the Laparoscopic Approach

Laparoscopy would always have a theoretical risk of dissemination of the parasite; this risk is compounded by the absence of the adequate measures that are taken in open surgery, such as the use of large surgical pads soaked in scolicidal agents (Hanan 2005; Malik et al. 2017). Adequate necessary precautions should be taken to avoid spillage during surgery, including the use of high-pressure suction devices, aspiration, and several irrigations of the cyst before extraction of the laminated membranes is done (Malik et al. 2017). Utmost care should be taken during the extraction of the laminated membrane and the daughter cysts to avoid any dissemination of the parasite. Endobags can be safely used for the extraction of the laminated membrane.

Recent Advances

Recently, robot-assisted surgical management of hydatid disease has been gaining attention.

References

Alper A, Emre A, Hazar H, Ozden I, Bilge O, Acarli K, et al. Laparoscopic surgery of hepatic hydatid disease: initial results and early follow-up of 16 patients. World J Surg. 1995;19:725–8.

Balik AA, Bmahmut M, et al. Surgical treatment of hydatid disease of liver—review of 304 cases. Arch Surg. 1999;134(2):166–9.

Bari S, Malik AA, Arif SH. Role of albendazole in the management of hydatid cyst liver. Saudi J Gastroenterol. 2011;17(5):343–7.

Baskaran V, Patnaik PK. Feasiblity and safety of laparoscopic management of hydatid disease of liver. JSLS. 2004;8:359–63.

Bhadreshwara KA, et al. Comparative study of laparoscopic versus open surgery. IAIM. 2015;2(1):30–5.

Bickel A, Eitan A. The use of a large, transparent cannula, with a beveled tip, for safe laparoscopic management of hydatid cysts of liver. Surg Endosc. 1995;9:1304–5.

Bickel A, Loberant N, Shtamler B. Laparoscopic treatment of cyst of the liver: initial experience with a small series of patients. J Laparoendosc Surg. 1994;4:127–33.

Bickel A, Loberant N, Singer-Jordan J, Goldfeld M, Daud G, Eitan A. The laparoscopic approach to abdominal hydatid cysts: a prospective nonselective study using the isolated hypobaric technique. Arch Surg. 2001;136:789–95.

Bilge A, Sozuer EM. Diagnosis and surgical treatment of hepatic hydatid disease. HPB Surg. 1994;8:77–81.

Busic Z, Cupurdija K, Servis D, et al. Surgical treatment of liver echinococcosis–open or laparoscopic surgery? Coll Antropol. 2012;36(4):1363–6.

Buttenschoen K, Carli Buttenschoen D. *Echinococcus granulosus* infection: the challenge of surgical treatment. Langenbecks Arch Surg. 2003;388:218–30.

Christian KK, Pitt HA. Hepatic abscess cystic disease of liver. In: Zinner MJ, Ashley SW, editors. Mangots abdominal operations. 11th ed. New York: McGraw Hill; 2007. p. 757–81.

Ertem M, Karahasanoglu T. Laparoscopically treated liver hydatid cysts. Arch Surg. 2002;137:1170–3.

Gupta N, Oza V, et al. Comparative study between laparoscopic versus open deroofing in 30 cases of liver hydatid cyst. IJSR. 2014;3(9):382–6.

Hanan R. Rihani et al. Laparoscopic approach to liver hydatid cyst. JRMS 2005;12(2):69–71.

Jauhari A, Golhar KB. Management of hepatic hydatidosis by laparoscopic approach in rural central India; A 3 year experience. Int J Res Med Sci. 2014;2:100–3.

Khoury G, Geagea T, Hajj A, et al. Laparoscopic treatment of hydatid cysts of the liver. Surg Endosc. 1994;8(9):1103–4 [PubMed].

Khuroo MS, Wani NA, Javid G, Khan BA, Yattoo GN, Shah AH, et al. Percutaneous drainage compared with surgery for hepatic hydatid cysts. N Engl J Med. 1997;337:881–7.

Malik AA, Ayoub I, Wani MA, Bari SU. Laparoscopic versus conventional surgery for hepatic hydatid disease: a comparative study. J Minim Invasive Surg Sci. 2017;6(4):e57109.

Mamarajabov S, Kodera Y, Karimov S, et al. Surgical alternatives for hepatic hydatid disease. Hep Gastroentrol. 2011;58:112.

Milicevic MN. Hydatid disease. In: Blumgart LH, Fong Y, editors. Surgery of the liver and biliary tract. 3rd ed. Philadelphia, PA: WB Saunders Company Ltd; 2002. p. 1167–204.

Rihani HR, et al. Laparoscopic approach to liver hydatid cyst. JRMS. 2005;12(2):69–71.

Rooh-ul-Muqim, Kamran K, Khalil J, Gul T, Farid S. Laparoscopic treatment of hepatic hydatid cyst. J Coll Physicians Surg Pak. 2011;21(8):468–71.

Saglam A. Laparoscopic treatment of liver hydatid cysts. Surg Laparosc Endosc. 1996;6:16–21.

Sayek I. Cystic hydatid disease: current trends in diagnosis and management. Surg Today. 2004;34(12):987–96.

Sayek I, Onat D. Diagnosis and treatment of uncomplicated hydatid cyst of the liver. World J Surg. 2001;25:21–7.

WHO. WHO/OIE manual on echinococcosis in humans and animals: A public health problem of global concern. In: Eckert J, Gemmell MA, Meslin FX, Pawlowski ZS, editors. Echinococcosis in humans: clinical aspects, diagnosis and treatment. Paris, France: OIE Publications; 2001. p. 20–66.

Zaharie F, Bartos D. Open or laparoscopic treatment for hydatid disease of the liver? A 10-year single-institution experience. Surg Endosc. 2013;27(6):2110–6.